Awakening To A New Mind

'Awakening To A New Mind' 1st edition.
Published by MetaVision Productions, Queensland, Australia.
Copyright © 2023 by MetaVision Pty Ltd.
Web Site: www.acosmicmind.com   Email: metavision37@gmail.com

Illustrator and Cover Designer - Margo Bobrowicz
Website: www.margobobrowicz

Supported Self-Publishing Author - MRW Publishing
coauthorbooks@gmail.com

All rights reserved. No part of this book may be reproduced in any form or by any means without permission in writing from the publisher.

The information within this book has been compiled by the author Luxor and Elle. While the opinions expressed herein are endorsed by the publisher, the publisher wishes to indemnify itself from any controversy that may arise as a result of misinterpretation or misunderstanding.

National Library of Australia Cataloguing-in-Publication
McAlpine, Bruce.
Awakening To A New Mind

1st ed.
Includes index.
ISBN
Paperback – 978 - 0 - 9580315 - 3 - 0
eBook – 978 - 0 - 9580315 - 2 - 3

1. Channelling (Spiritualism). 2. Guides (Spiritualism).
3. Angels - Miscellanea. I. Title.
133.9

Testimonials

Awakening to a New Mind is a highly recommended read with its core focus on gaining a greater understanding of the ultimate question "Who We Are". It provides a peaceful calming effect to what is currently happening in world affairs today as it paints a broader picture of what is more important to focus on, which is the journey into the fifth dimension.

Paul Luxford

Within the hidden cells of the human psyche there is waiting to be revealed a new mind and memory, which stands ready to inspire a methodical manner of living free, an advanced way of greeting providence, with a timely preparation for understanding and engaging future eventualities. Reading an 'Awakening to a New Mind' offers that opportunity.

Nikki Knights

Awakening to a New Mind is a fascinating writing style that explores in depth, the awakening to the Fifth Dimension, identified cosmically as the new sphere of existence as we know it.

The theory of the Fifth Dimension was conceived by Swedish physicist Oskar Klein, as a dimension unseen by humans where the forces of gravity and electromagnetism unite to create a simple but graceful theory of the fundamental forces. 5D beings can oscillate themselves through the spiritual and physical world and understand the spiritual laws of the universe.

MetaVision takes the reader on a journey that begins with the transformation from the acceptance that our basic understanding of the valued aim of society is for people to survive, to one the authors explain as their cosmic interest being inherent in people coming alive!

Tracy Tully MRW Publishing

Are you prepared for the dawning of a New Day and a New Mind? In Awakening to a New Mind, the reader is introduced to the prediction that planet Earth and its human beings as we know it, are heading towards a gigantic shake up of planetary reorganisation.

The present-day confusion, pressure and turbulence in mind and memory that we witness daily, has been revealed internationally as the forerunners to a celestial reorganisation.

The gift of the Fifth Dimension is that every human child born into planetary life today, has the potential to access cosmic awareness.

Terressa Elliott

In the position of cosmic pioneers, the authors of Awakening to a New Mind offer a newfound understanding of worth as a measure of strength in foundation.

Explanations so far given on life mysteries are like working on a jigsaw puzzle that has central pieces missing.

These Cosmic pioneers guide a greater understanding into entering a fulfilled life of improved Health, increased Wealth, and building enduring relationships with appealing qualities such as connection and engagement.

Lisa Burney

When the Two worlds Merge

Man marches eternally
To the timeless beat of drum
Yet Love is beyond
Awakened memories
Connect a self with self
No longer duality
The door to Home is open

In a state of nothingness there is stillness
Silence composed of a beautiful sound
Where cosmic colours are illustrated
Music of the spheres is orchestrated

Dedication to the Great Mother

Our dedication and devotion, first and foremost, is to the Great Mother, the purveyor of female energy in the embrace of Love.

In our time spent in planetary fields and our background forming from cosmic fields, we wish to give due consideration to Angel energy. Angels on behalf of Mother Energy watch over us benignly. Angels have given us consideration for our future benefit in acknowledgement of our dedication. They are our friends.

These stories, explanations, and metaphysical discourses are listed as a series of book essays written in response to Greater Energy entities who have cosmically fashioned the lives of planetary humans and other like species within the dimensional spaces of the cosmos dating back at least two and a half million years.

Love, wisdom, and understanding of beauty include the principles of **Truth**, **Equality**, and **Unity** as proposed by the One. The ability to interpret and develop certain necessary portions of what is called the Divine Plan extends far beyond the limitations of rational thinking; especially beliefs still being exercised by august people on this planet: specifically those who see themselves as the last word on all matters philosophical, religious, or scientific.

Dedication by Lucifer Energy

Unto the Great Mother energy, she who emerged fully formed from the waves of the Great Ocean, humans owe their very existence. From her first born, known as The One, people have received the beneficial factors of progressive understanding into the present day.

When the cosmic morrow, referenced as the New Day appears, people will take to heart the endorsement of the Great Mother Love. The dawning light heralds in the approaching Fifth Dimension. People will participate in a makeover from estrangement into a new arrangement.

First there comes the breaking down of old patterns, errant beliefs, those religious innuendos fashioned and hardened by the rigorous efforts of moral indignation, ordered and incoordinated by male authority.

The wily ruses employed by society rulers to command obedience from unwitting subjects on the planet is soon to be declared null and void.

Coterie of Players

Luxor and Jézel acknowledge those whom we serve, those who cosmically oversee our work areas and service the Greater Good.

We take our working instructions from the wishes of the Great Mother.

We take counsel from the One, the Unnamed, and the Great Dragon who are incorporated with the Greater Council of Nine. Other members have included the Los Diabolos, Shining Ones, and Lords of Lightning who have in recent times merged into the Greater Energy.

We take advisement from the Angels who work on behalf of the Line of Mothers and Love energy.

We have camaraderie with Jésu, Charlie, and any amount of like entity/energies who serve the Greater Energy while roaming through the vastness of galaxies.

We are conversant with the WE Energy that is beyond memory.

We are familiar with Ancients who were the architects and builders of the universal system and Elementals who assisted in providing the fauna and flora decorating the planets.

Sataan – a mentor of Lucifer and organizer of the landing of the 37 on planet Earth.

October 2016

After dinner, we move to the lounge room where Jézel goes into channel mode.

Beyond Messenger: The message comes from far back. There are dark days that lie ahead for this planet Earth, all consuming, all dark. However, what we would like you to regard is that what is abstract will become identifiable, will become obvious. That which has been locked in a negative frame or picture for eons will become manifest. This is for you to observe, regard, and notify as pioneering scribes of these historic events as they are happening today. Humans are not up to speed in understanding global circumstances. They are several paces behind.

For ye who are involved and devoted to the greater energy, specifically the Great Mother energy, you will act as co-ordinators and journalists of historic…they are not considered historic yet as they are still futuristic…but they will be historic events as they occur.

Well, this may all appear enigmatic when you type it out, read it out, but eventually a bigger picture will become clear to you. The negative imprint will in the near future start to become obvious.

We are imparting this to you because we understand that you are and will be cognisant with this next chapter, not only in the history of this planet, but also of the cosmic arena as well.

You have our heartfelt, womb-felt feelings move into you this evening. Thank you.

Involvement

*I do not know how not to love you
This human bondage which we share
Though driven crazy with despair
Has compensations while the true
Self needing nothing is reviled
The false tarted for pleasure has beguiled
Human common sense. What has left
The body leaves the mind bereft*

*When caught in meditative state
Nothing is quite what it seems
We pause to consider our sad fate
Being locked within our dreams*

*The rhythm of pulse stirs memories
Not of this world. Beyond, above
Lies another land of mysteries
Calling us home to a Mother's love*

This We Pledge

We Are Aligned With Who We Represent

As devoted and dedicated children to the Great Mother, we are working in service to the Greater Energy. We have been nominated cosmically as lost children, yet with what we have come to understand in recent times we consider we are no longer lost.

Who are we? That is the question each person is required to ask of their selves. Given that we are prodigies of Greater Energy sent forth with roles to play out on this planet Earth is it necessary that we should know the answer to the question? Or is the answer to the question simply to respond that we are in planetary appearance no one special. In effect we are projections of Greater Energy. We exist to use our planetary being for the benefit of developing a greater understanding of Love and Intelligence to be shared globally amongst tribal societies without discrimination.

In fact our cosmic roles on planet Earth are to ignite the energy fires of Love and Intelligence, which in turn will return missing elements of communal welfare into the arms and bosom of the Great Mother. Then in respect for her wisdom and beauty, we will involve and mentally embrace each other through absorbing the greater understanding incorporating Love energy. Thus far we are small in numbers; however, our efforts in motivating human delivery into returning Home are designed to be witnessed as great. Our wishes in serving the Great Mother are beyond the wasted hopes of so many seeing themselves as superior in the operative planetary systems.

****

Our immediate purpose is to complete the elongated curve between cosmos and planet Earth, meaning this journey already undertaken, will complete through going full circle into wholeness.

Our role on this planet today is mainly to ingest the minds of awakening people with the benefit of greater understanding. It is role-playing for us to divest others of what are wasted beliefs and then introduce new levels of Cosmic Intelligence. It is not our area to promote Love as such. Love energy will develop its own platforms for awakening the enclosed hearts. It will create its own level of fullness. We are not here to be seen as deliverers of Love, per example.

Our work is to step out momentarily from the absorption of Love Energy and by such means available introduce to people a greater understanding of Love. Though we can say we come from Love, which we do, it does not mean that we are to exude Love as such. For Love does not have need of proponents. Love exists within Love. So though we can say we are born of Love, which we are, we do not wish to demonstrate Love in planetary form or style.

What we can demonstrate are the areas that Love has decreed to be opened and developed; such as wisdom, beauty, and Intelligence provisioning methods for greater understanding. All of these are children of Love energy. Or, if you prefer, they are an exponential evolution of Love energy. As such, in obedience to the Great Mother whom we acknowledge as the female expansion of Love, we are her devoted children.

On a greater scale you might say that that is not exactly how life is to be seen, but we are not interested in working on that greater scale. What we are interested in doing is working within the arms of the Great Mother, so that the work we do on this planet echoes her brilliance, which is declared as wisdom, beauty, style, and grace.

So let's not get ourselves over excited about saying, 'oh, we can go back beyond that because we know that that was not the beginning'. Within ourselves we can have a small understanding of that, but if that is where we want to push a barrow then we will deny the area of work we have been put on this planet to develop. So we are all for obeying the wishes of the Great Mother.

Let others tell us that Love has its place, and no doubt in their visionary platforms they see a greater picture. That is not our concern. We were born to embrace life and observe the face of the Great Mother. We are not here to proclaim the be all and end all of human greatness, or of its intended cosmic fellowship.

We each have a role to play. We have beauty to observe within and then bring forth into light a display of its magnificence. We have a life to live and we have the concepts of living free to bring into prominence an effect that is still shrouded by a dreaming state. That is an indication of our gifted roles; that is a small glimpse of our future work areas. In duty bound we will observe the necessary steps and so make the shifts in future happenings occur as smoothly as possible for humankind.

We love that which we are born to be part of. We do not question whatever the overall picture happens to be demonstrating. It is enough for us to know that we are working arduously as functionaries of Love energy.

We have access to cosmic Intelligence, and that which we carry we share to inform others of their cosmic birthright. The overall effect is going to enhance the livelihood of every being on planet Earth. This we solemnly pledge.

Contents

Foreword i
   Introduction to a New Day & a New Mind i

Chapter I. The Great Ocean and Great Mother 1
   The Great Ocean 1
   Introducing the Great Mother 5
   Love as Energy 6

Chapter II. Building of the Universe 10
   Early Cosmic Settlements 10
   Causing of the Solar System 11
   Setting the Record Straight 12
   Initial Birthing of Planet Earth 15

Chapter III. Angels 21
   Walking and Talking in Harmony with Angels 21
   Observation 24
   The Messenger 24

Chapter IV. The Divine Family 27
   Arrival on Earth - The Divine Family 28
   Question Time at the Table 34
   The Landing of the 37 37

Chapter V. The Cosmic Twins 45
   Discussion 48
   Birthing of Lucifer 48
   Christos Light 53
   Lucifer Experience 55
   Discussion with Jésu and Lucifer 56

Chapter VI. Greater Council of Nine 70
   Discussion with the Greater Council of Nine 70
   Discussion with an Envoy of the Great Dragon 76
   Discussion with the Great Dragon 81
   Discussion with the Great Dragon 83

Chapter VII. Cosmic Energy 85
   Discussion with the Greater Energy 85
   A Second Visit from the Greater Lucifer 90
   Discussion with Callers of the Shots 91
   Discussion with Illustrious Ones 97
   Discussion with Colour & Sound - 1 99
   Discussion with Colour & Sound – 2 103

Chapter VIII. Fifth Dimension & New Day 106
- Dawning of the New Day 107
- Recovery and Discovery 109
- Shift to the 5th Dimension 110
- Fifth Dimension Discourse 111
- Spiritual Development 112
- The Hollow Arena 113
- A Sitting in the Hollow Arena 114
- Showcase 117

Chapter IX. A Cosmic Mind 122
- Introduction 123
- Promoting the New Mind and Brain 124
- A Well-Kept Mind 126
- Locating the Essential Oil Within 127
- The Product 129
- Three in One 130
- Converting Three Diversities into One 131
- Health Wealth & Relationship 132
- Psyche 133
- Smashing the Mirrors 135
- Reflected Glory 136
- Mirror Visualization 137

Chapter X. Love & Intelligence 139
- Awakening into the Light 140
- Love Intelligence & the Great Ocean 141
- The Carpet & its Design 143
- Intelligence 143
- Becoming Mentally Aware 146
- Love is Energy 149
- Where is Foundation 152
- Love is All 155

Chapter XI. Two Selves 157
- Getting to Know You Series 158
- Who and what are the Two Selves 161
- Reconnection of Essence and Presence 162
- Preference for Essence 164
- Inner Self Work 166

Chapter XII. Our Background & Work 168
- Cosmic Pioneers 169
- Breaking through Outmoded Barriers 173
- Background Sketch of Discovery 174
- Experimental work in the Psyche 176

Chapter XIII. Lucifer Essays 179
    The Call Within 180
    If You have a Light, Shine It 183
    Iconic Gods with Clay Feet 183
    Human Heritage 186

Chapter XIV. Epilogue 190
    Summary 191

Chapter XV. Preview of 'The Star Within' 193
    The Future of Womanhood 193
    The Rainbow Trail 195

Table of Poems

The Fantasy in Love	4
The Hidden Wells of Life	19
Veil of the Mother	27
The Song of 37	37
Oh, Wretched Being	45
Going Home	51
Indomitable Spirit	68
Remembering	84
Dawning of the New Day	106
A Cosmic Awakening	122
Love is All	139
That Love is All	155
Cup of Life	156
On Meeting Strangers	157
Two Genies	164
We are Almost There	168
There is No God	179
A Need In Deed to Know	189
Wondrous Events	192
Being-in-Love	196

Foreword

Introduction to a New Day & a New Mind

The Book of Life, which is eternal, has no set beginnings. Yet each chapter in the book that we identify with offers the opportunity for a new approach in mind and spirit to access a greater understanding of loving and living freely.

Each chapter in 'Awakening to a New Mind' delivers a cosmic presentation concerning the progression of human life and the prospect of living free of present day planetary fixations in minds that are erroneous. These essays are an advent purposefully composed to welcome into mind and memory the incoming Fifth Dimension.

The following material has been compiled from discussions with beyond entity/energies of cosmic distinction, those who make their existence known to us through mental exchanges and verbal forms of channelled discussion. The translations make use of the English language and have been consistent in the same delivered style that began more than 25 years ago.

A major theme in communications with specific regard to this planet references a backlog of incidents that happened in the corridors of the Cosmos eons ago. Were it to be measured in linear time the record of related events would span some three million years and more.

The discussions occur between characters cosmically situated and even some further beyond with those of us who are strategically placed to activate human awareness on planet Earth. We are required to narrate the exchanges between worlds of dimensional difference. These dialogues for human interest and advancement have been duly recorded and filed as the saying goes for future reference. This third dimensional atmosphere is losing its walled in strength of denial and Earth is being welcomed into a new chapter of cosmic existence duly noted as the Fifth Dimension.

We speak regularly and extensively with entity/energies that exist in the various dimensional levels where they have an overview on most things planetary with regard to its future usefulness. Recently though, many of the exchanges have been reduced to mental directives that guide our understandings without spoken passages.

We do not expect that the majority of people on the planet today are going to readily embrace the greater communiqués of Love energy and Intelligence being proposed for their future welfare, nor accepting without murmur the credibility of characters interviewed and reviewed to be openly received and accepted for the benefit of all. What we can say though is the proof of the pudding is in the eating. Those who take time out to digest that which is freely imparted will benefit accordingly.

The essays compiling some of the historic journeys of interplay energy between cosmos and planets do not claim to be totally accurate in planetary time or space travel. What is written and offered for public consideration are extracts taken from the main thrust of purposeful deliveries for the benefit of awakening and advancing humankind. The explanations offer fresh information beyond recorded knowledge for those interested in a greater awareness of human existence and proposed future events.

Certainly the intention in the exercising of a new mind is to fill in some of the clouded gaps that have deluded the unwitting enterprises of philosophy, science, and religious side-tracking that have led people on the planet off course for long periods of time. The sequential incidents that were played out in early times extend far beyond the recall of present day human memory.

Enough to say that those entity/energies who now speak in various ways to inform people who take time out to stop and listen are not suffering from the maladies still haunting the minds and souls of the many; those who have inherited the present day faulty ideas of religion and science that muddle and befuddle human consciousness.

Foreword

Unnamed One: Throughout the varying stages of planet Earth recovery some of us who were original members of the cosmic coded 37 return to continue the work of upgrading human sensibilities. One of our varied tasks is to release the latent or somnolent minds from the ongoing drag of reptilian and limbic memories that linger. To further advance human mentality beyond the neo-cortex jumble of fixated ego thinking, that which erroneously declares certain races are more entitled than others to be masters of this empirical existence.

****

Initially the code-named 37 were formed as an elite corps of cosmic agents, known as star runners, sent to explore and pull planet Earth from its third dimensional plunge back into the Cosmos Proper from whence it went hurtling into separation mode some two and a half million years ago.

Being cast into the roles of cosmic drop-ins or walk-ins we periodically enter into approved human bodies as dedicated cosmic workers offering our services once more to pursue the designs of Greater Energy; those who are situated to work beyond the limited cosmic fields of stars and planets. We number amongst those who are involved in promoting the features of the Divine Plan as a prelude to the opening of an even Greater Plan for the further benefit of rearranging the futures of myriad cosmic families.'

A portion of the workload that involves us is to speak for the advancement of a greater understanding of Life and living free of argument as a means to release the resident human presence on Earth; where people are still locked down, trapped in illusionary mental states of a misguided third dimensional professed reality.

****

The material we offer for consideration is written to jog the memories of half a million cosmic entities, loosely called Angelics, who are presently residing on planet Earth in various guises of human formation. They are required to become responsibly awakened and aware of whom they really are, whom they cosmically represent, and commit to the planetary tasks of future human development they agreed to perform eons ago.

Many of them have already been partially awakened only to become enmeshed in empirical and universal garbage defined as profit taking.

They have been sucked into a swampland wallow by fourth dimensional programs that only make a pretence at dispensing love and light.

****

To open up a greater understanding of being as revealed today we first must go back to the circumstances that caused the building of the surrounding planets in the universe energised by the star energy Ra and the setting up of seven planets that still occupy portions of its initial orbital space.

Following on from that disclosed information we invite the world to meet with members of the Divine Family and others responsible for the introduction of planets Earth and Venus, who took up their relative roles to further the exposition of the Divine Plan.

This book is more expansive in cosmic understanding than our previous book, 'The Gift of the Rose', being organized and written 21 years later, though some parts are inclusive and make reference to earlier material. We introduce more graphically the members of the **Divine Family, Angels.** and other notable characters and groupings such as the **Greater Council of Nine**, reflecting their differing roles as they have an influence on the development and implementation of the homeward journey that engages Earth and its varied species of human elementals.

We are pleased to introduce **The Great Mother** who responsibly overviews the development of **Divine Womanhood** destined to become the next featured role of female leadership on planet Earth.

Chapter I.

The Great Ocean and Great Mother

The Great Ocean

Every droplet of water, albeit in streamlet, creek, or river, once set in motion remorselessly leads us likewise into a stream of greater cosmic understanding that is taking us Home, into the Great Ocean from whence our energy was first formed.

We are advised we are Love-in-being so we are eternal in spirit. People on planet Earth are on a journey back home to the cosmos proper to rediscover who they are. We have come from the waves of the Great Ocean and we are returning home by predestined procedure. Some have called it the journey back to the future.

When the light of consciousness split the darkness of the great oceanic depths beyond linear time and memory the living energy of the Great Mother emerged and gave birth to the One. With that arrival from essence Intelligence came into an awareness of understanding self as a being of interest. Presence is a term we use for attained human consciousness, but it is only half of a picture. We are subject to the One, which is a descriptive term of an energy source of comprehensive understanding that pervades and overviews the vastness of those at work in cosmic fields.

The designation of **Truth, Equality, and Unity** were posited as first principles of Intelligence promoted from the One. In this manner of giving access to levels of greater understanding for the benefit of those with receptive minds, there is offered an elemental formation of brilliant light deriving from the essence of Love.

Truth, Equality, and **Unity** *are the principled symbols offered by the One.* There is equality in accepting all living things as being fellow creatures. Unity arrives in knowing that all things are enjoining as one. Truth that surrounds and abounds realizes and encompasses the demonstration of beauty in all.

Each and every one of us who carry routine lines of Love and Intelligence within ourselves have had it initially born through the delivery of the Great Mother energy that rose into being from out of the depths of the Great Ocean. And that being the case, when we return to Home base as we are required to do at the completion of our cosmic journeying, it will be to enter into the arms of the Great Mother and then to rest once more in the allotted deep of the Great Ocean.

13th May 2015

The Great Mother: This planetary world that you are involved in is fast losing its opportunity to create a spiralling effect. We, and I don't just speak of myself when I use that word, are all for spiralling. But it would seem that there is a necessity for a downward effect to occur before the new stage or phase of development will be acknowledged and appreciated. Therefore we have advised each of you to spiral downwards because we have said to you and will say to you again that you have to find your foundation in the depths of the Great Ocean.

****

The Great Ocean is the purveyor of all feeling. People of science talk with authority about the motion of tidal waves, but the stressed movement from the internal sea that humans have labelled emotions is simply the surface level of what can be seen as obvious, being similar in turmoil to the white caps on the ocean waves about to break asunder on the shoreline. The unrealized currents of feeling residing within the great ocean are immersed in its depths. So in similar fashion is the human system ascribed to the playground of the elements.

Thus joy is deeper within the human system than token displays of happiness. People lap up a surface layer of happiness like a kitten whose eyes have not fully opened tackles a bowl of milk. When people of the planet finally come awake they will realise that the happiness they previously sought was simply a small foaming flurry on top of a deeper wave of energy, a smattered covering overlaying a deeper stretching pressure of becoming aware or awake in greeting the enlightenment of a New Day.

28th August 2014

The One: Okay, listen up! So the foundation of all life, happenings, experience, is Love. Then from that Love, if you see it like a stem of the flower, it is competent to produce a floribunda of blooms. And what are those blooms? There is Intelligence, then there is Wisdom, there is Beauty, and further to those areas there is Style and Grace, which are the personifications of Divine Womanhood.

Other blossoms have produced Intelligence. They have produced the three principles, **Truth**, **Equality**, and **Unity**. And none of these blooms that we speak of are meant to remain as unopened flowers. So it is with this work that is to be performed on the planet, the requirement is to see these blooms blossoming forth.

Who is it that speaks with you this evening? I have been nominated as the One. The first child to be born of the Great Mother energy. And yes, Intelligence is my forte. However, I am competent to speak of the various roles of Wisdom, Beauty, Style and Grace, and of course, the three principles that I have pronounced as **Truth**, **Equality**, and **Unity**.

Outside of these there are many areas that are extensions of what is already stated…I wish I could say understanding, but on a planetary level of course they are far from being understood. So it is our work as the children, in which I include myself, of the Great Mother, to make these understandings comprehensible to humans.

****

Luxor: So let us go from the introduction of the **One** unto the three principles, which are nominated as the basic accord for finding balance in all life practices. Each time that the elements or the energy drop into another level so then the three principles of **Truth**, **Equality**, and **Unity** are required to drop accordingly. So no matter how far that you move through the essentials, through the dimensional levels, be it the association with One, be it cosmos, be it universal, planetary, sub-planetary, those three elements, those three principles, are as magnificently measured as they were from the very first moment of existence.

No one can alter in any way, shape, or form, the principled essence of **Truth**, **Equality**, and **Unity**. They are solid, they are sound, and they are inextricably valid. So in all of our actions, in all of our ideas of how we can demonstrate a particular style, the only way that we can remain valid is that we are bonded by dedication to the three principles.

The Fantasy in Love

(Dedicated to the Great Mother)

I have seen the thoughtful look
Gazed enrapt into green eyes
Felt the burn of strong small hands
Joined with her in ringing laughter
Sat soft and quiet by still water
Trapped by rocks. The very last
Of waters that flowed in times long past

Red rust of flowers, green sward of leaves
What strange fantasy each spell weaves
Images resembling stained glass windows
Set in tall cathedrals. The breeze blows
Birds may sing or give out chatter
Turtles plop and lizards scatter
None of this is of much matter
Love is All plays out mystery
That beckons and engages me
I have little will, even less choice
I still tremble when I hear her voice

Introducing the Great Mother

27th April 2012

The Great Mother is the womb of life from whence comes all creative activity.

Great Mother: Come to ME, oh my children, those I sent forth to bear my wishes. Return unto the hearth where the arms of the Great Mother bids you welcome. The times of pain and pressure are ending and what we always foresaw is now in nature blending. You are ME. Never more nor less. Our work was ever to address that which hope offered to redress, but could not attain while the foolishness was 'god bless'. So I say again, come to ME, my children. Our house is empty until your joyous clamour fills our hearts with the noise of your return.

4th November 2013

Lucifer: Who can say that they have a call on Love energy? Who can say they have a call on Intelligence? Who can say that they have the last word in wisdom, beauty, style, and grace? In which case then we are all learners, novices, tyros, small children of the Great Mother let loose on planet Earth to access a greater understanding of being.

When are we prepared to sit at her feet in front of the fireplace and listen to her tell us the stories of where we have come from, reassure us of where we are at, and advise us as to where we are meant to be advancing? When we can take that lode on board then we are competent to represent the wishes of the Great Mother. But while we remain in our petulant states of arrogance that wants to tell the Great Mother we have got a bigger handle on understanding living arrangements without the benefit of her wisdom we continue to demonstrate the ignorant and arrogant state of lost children.

There is nothing wrong with the demonstration of the child. It is recommended that we go back to that position or situation regularly. But if your pride and your arrogance say that you are an advance on that which is conveyed then you are in a state of mental kerfuffle. Jésu said when they asked him, 'how would they be admitted into understanding the kingdom of heaven' he replied, 'become the child'.

Two thousand years later nothing much has altered. If you wish to be admitted into what has been nominated as the kingdom of heaven…we don't agree with the wording of the title, though we do agree with the state you will only arrive through becoming the child. The child that is required to sit at the feet of the Great Mother.

The Great Mother is not as you might imagine her as a Great Mother. That, if you like, is a conundrum because your human idea of a great mother is not how the Great Mother represents. The Great Mother is wholeness. She is male and she is female. She is beyond any level or idea of conception that you might carry. In other words, to say what you consider the Great Mother is will sell yourself short because her energy is beyond comprehension. So to buy an idea of the Great Mother you only weaken yourself internally because she is more than any conclusion.

We who are her children are bonded into her energy. And in that energy field there is no such thing as description. In her arms you have no past. You have no present. You are without future. You are simply bonded into greater energy. And it does not matter what happens to you on this planet. The best that you can do on this planet is to work on behalf of the Great Mother. The worst you can do is denying the worth in your own beauty. The joy in living free is in becoming full or totally whole.

There is no tomorrow. That may sound incongruous because surely today has to step into another form of location. Tomorrow is actually derived from yesterday. Each one of us sitting in this room this evening, along with some who are not here tonight, is a blessed child of the Great Mother. All we ask is that when you read the material you take cognisance of yourself and in doing so endorse the wishes of the Great Mother.

Love as Energy

Love as female energy nominated as the Great Mother moved through an endless flow of nothingness to mate with the eternal connection and in so doing gave birth to The One, thus forming Intelligence, which kinetically appeared as a spiral of flaming energy. Intelligence in turn projected for the sake of utility three principles of kinetic energy known cosmically as **Truth**, **Equality**, and **Unity**.

These three are noted principles so they are not set into visible form as actualities. In realization there is a requirement for a greater understanding than any rational mind can glean from knowledge defined as scholarly types of education. The easiest method of demonstrating an understanding of Love energy and its principles is through a mix of analogy and allegory.

So let us see Truth like the ingredients necessary for the baking of a cake. We put into a bowl the measured quantities to ensure the correct mix of Equality. Then we stir the ingredients to a smooth mixture and this instils Unity. Bake the cake at a suitable temperature, which we call balance, and when it cools make sure you sample its quality first before extending the fare to others. Only when we are satisfied in the quality of the taste should we feel free to share it with others.

Humans stand in Truth and because of that positioning cannot see the bigger picture of life that surrounds them. Truth is always available for us to draw down the understandings that provide the necessities of planetary living. Equality is finding the balance between those things that touch and affect our very being. Unity is mixing, melding and moulding until we are blended into a shapely level of quality allowance. When these functions are achieved the baking moves into a further art form called acceptance.

The finished product that is then required to be consumed is Love energy.

Someone once wrote that love makes the world go round. This world that humans occupy was designed and built by energies in the Cosmos Proper we call the Ancients. Venus was built by the instruction of the Divine Mother to act in part as a support system for planet Earth and followed its entry into the universal spin called atmosphere. That support is still in progress today.

A planet like any other thing that can be envisioned comes from a wish, a desire for fulfilment of some purpose. Reason and purpose are not the same. Desire comes from beyond the mind. When it enters the mind for the purpose of exposure it becomes an urge. It acts as an irritation. The irritation activates as a drive to create a measure of fulfilment.

Fulfilment is not the whole picture. Development does not complete a picture. It creates a cameo of relationships in life. The human world is a cameo piece set in a bigger cosmic picture. Humans are nurtured by the energy of Love and are ministered by cosmic workers referred to as Angels.

When humans can move beyond the idea that the frames they view are corporeal in substance only and nothing more, then they will be ready to come out of kindergarten status and have access to cosmic levels of intelligence, where the ego sense no longer dominates planetary thinking. The 'my' and the 'I am' are featured as pride of self-ownership and no more than delusions of the egocentric child obsessed with a reflection of its own image.

Does the child want to know from where it derives its energy? Does it question its own existence? Not seriously. It will settle for bedtime stories built by religions and socially acceptable material delivered from media platforms that churn out mental pap with monotonous regularity. The human ego regardless of age is a childlike creature who does not question so long as the food it requires for nourishment appears regularly on demand. We are using food in a wider context of personal satisfaction.

There are galaxies existent beyond human comprehension teeming with intelligent life. There are planets in this solar system loaded with beings with far more advanced levels of civilisation than humanity. All of which the scientific leadership on Earth, wrapped in cocoons of their own ego importance, are oblivious to and refer to all such developed interacting material as science fiction. When it suits them what they decry as fictitious today science will when given the opportunity promote the same as their established forms of truth tomorrow.

This Earth is a planet of people naming and labelling. If anything can be labelled then it can be separated, categorized and stored without requiring further examination. By stored we mean mentally boxed. There is a double whammy in this world of duality. What is boxed by the boxer retains and contains the shadow mind of the boxer.

These are painful lessons yet to be learned. One would think that anyone with common sense when they catch hold of something too hot to handle would be only too happy to release it. Not so the rational mind. Compulsively it grasps at whatever is too painful to hold in memory. It is besotted with containing pain. Pain is a temporary fix for those deprived of innate feeling. Deprivation in turn breeds depravity.

The juicy slugs of wickedness and corruption that feed off religious morality come into play. We repeat that the rational mind is obsessed with fear and pain. It is fixated with causes. Following the leader is a game for the likes of immature children. When will the sycophantic humans find their feet instead of crawling and grovelling after those they see as more advantaged or superior creatures?

Small children cannot help but see their parents as godlike figures and their teddy bears as friends. At some stage there will be a requirement for the children to stack the toys, say goodbye to the teddies and ask the parents whether there is anything they can do to assist in a restoration of social harmony. At that moment of awareness the human child enters into the cosmic world of family instead of planetary fantasy.

At a greater level of consciousness your cosmic family waits to greet you. The Divine Family was deliberately placed into the cosmos proper to relate a greater understanding of life and living arrangement to benefit humanity. Part of their role playing is to give a lead in elevating the lives of humans.

Therefore we carry certain gifted roles and attributes, which are required to be played out through these shifting times we call subject to sequential timing. It is an inevitable circumstance that linear time is in its last stages of appearance and will disappear as a method of counting down the days in a few short years.

Chapter II.

Building of the Universe

Early Cosmic Settlements

Long ago, so distant that it is doubtful if any cosmic records still exist, a density of atmospheric pressures caused a loss of memory and identity to occur in some of the star energies pioneering areas of darkness that human science might nominate as unexplored space. This circumstance severed much of the connection with the support systems set in place by the builders of the cosmic systems.

The energy of Love was still filtering through and available to the lost pioneers, but not being easily recognizable there was a slow build up of a denial of heritage in the process of mind forgetting past events. This caused a separation that bred a dread of loneliness, a fearful pressure, which mentally formed into a requirement for protection. The isolated entities drifted even further away from their links with cosmic unity. In an attempt to maintain a standard of support for the separation they assumed was real, but could not fathom, they formed what came to be known as the Confederation of Star Energies.

They can be seen as a number of breakaway groups that became dissident in their attitudes towards the core energy because as their solitude increased it degenerated their memories and resulted in mistaken forms of separation.

With their expansionary overview of life what became obvious to the builders of these planetary existences was that in some way each of these particular star wagons had lost the equivalent of a wheel. To the lost and lonely settlers in star systems that provided little sustenance, and even less memory contact, a paranoia of loss was building, which caused them to think that whatever they surveyed was there of necessity to be possessed.

Some small thread within them suggested that this was not their prime purpose in seeking, but the needs of the fearful mind cried out for recognition so they began a credo of moral rectitude to justify an ownership of what they could grab. They developed methods of control that were pyramidal in design because in their weakened state of memory truth was fast becoming half-truths and the diamond, symbolic of Love energy, was reduced in size to a small triangle of third dimensional laws because of the narrow focus.

The Ancient builders scratched their version of what humans call heads and went back to the drawing boards to rewrite previous conclusions.

Causing of the Solar System

Through the intelligence systems utilized to observe galactic formations, some of the Ancients in the Cosmos Proper were made aware that the various developments of the planetary areas were not as on course as the promoters of the Divine Plan requested as required. When this information was debated within a general council forum some proposed a method they considered would be a quick-fix way of rectifying any sort of out of balance situations. These Ancients wanted to take a short cut approach towards remedying what seemed to be an ever increasing problem of cosmic memory loss.

They considered a portion of the Divine Plan should be temporarily pre-empted. They wanted a suspension of the part that referred to the sovereignty of each area having an overbearing say in the method of determining its future destiny. Their proposal amounted to much the same as what is being called pre-emptive military strikes on planet Earth today. It is called the option of exercising free will without question and gives the right of control to those who carry the most power to bust into and dominate any area they do not consider is secured for future events suited to their liking.

Their idea was to put the Divine Plan temporarily on hold and go through each diffident planet with a mopping up exercise and not worry about the devastating consequences. Having reached a concession point in their favour they then could go back to clean up and reform the areas. So it was put on the table to a full meeting of the Ancients, which was something like a United Nations forum, and it did not get agreement.

Then the suggestion was put forward that as there could not be a general agreement on the problem they should experiment with a portion of space that was basically unoccupied. All space is occupied in varying degrees of energy. Therefore it is a question of the varying levels of the energies in the space as to whether it could be utilized for experimentation or not.

If we were to go to a deserted area with the intention to build a new enterprise, humans may not be there, but there would be all kinds of reptiles, animal life, etc. So environmentally the area is occupied. However, it depends on the density of the area or how primitive it is as to whether the invading development would be seen as more beneficial.

The area or space where the Universe exists now, this solar system as deployed around the star energy of Ra, was occupied. It was not empty space. There were resident energies though not of any great significance. The Ancients therefore utilized the area to put into place a trial solar system with the agreement of the Shining Ones. Around the installation of Ra as the energy centre certain designated Ancients built approximately seven planets, each in their own particular image.

Setting the Record Straight

So then with the support of the Shining Ones, the Ancients of male oriented energy built the solar systems or cosmic wheels forming the observable planetary bodies in what science calls the Universe. They were aided by Angel energy and nature forces called Elementals. The solar hubs, called stars and suns, such as Ra, were programmed and set in place from the energy of the Shining Ones. They are not subject to the planning areas or the building of planets supervised in the main by Ancients and partly administered by Angels.

The Ancients ingested the planets with projections of their particular energy most prominently being Satan (Saturn), Zeus (Jupiter), Uranus and Neptune. With the assistance of Mars, Mercury and Pluto these seven planets then started up systems of free will, choice, do whatever you like syndromes. Basically it was like a system of piracy with a veil of privacy. The planets were placed into the solar system and they kicked the proverbial ball around with very few holds barred.

Each planet carries a persona relative to the energy responsible for its universal formation mirrored from its own likeness. Just like a strawberry plant. The mother plant sends out a vine that establishes a sucker and it is fed by the mother energy until it has found its own strength and then the feeder line withers and drops off. It is similar to the umbilical cord that supports the young embryo until the baby can emerge to find its own sustenance.

Two of the main energies were Zeus and Sataan known as Satan on planet Earth. Both have been described in Greek mythology though the energy of Saturn or Satan was more commonly known as Kronos, the marker of time. That particular line of energy still carries through its role. He maintains the clock of sequential timing that determines the ongoing destiny of planet Earth and the movement of its creatured people.

Zeus in mythology was the personality or projection of the planet Jupiter. In the greater picture it is shown clearly that Jupiter is an offshoot of Zeus. At that time Earth was not here or there because it was still in the design stages being nurtured in the cosmos proper. Neither was Venus.

In part the planets are experimental stations, including nurseries for new growth projects. On behalf of the Divine Mother the projected mankind was fashioned under the supervision of Sataan and the species of man were then assigned to populate planet Earth. The Sataan energy was also responsible for devising the previous planetary formation of Saturn.

The formula or design for Earth was built in the Cosmos Proper, which is a metropolis formed of cosmic entities representing distinctive strains of energies emanating from further beyond areas of understanding. In this manner they could observe the portions of what it was they carried within and give them the opportunity of rectifying any faults that required attention.

The climactic changes to the surface of the planet after it entered the solar system and settled into the third dimension cycle required an ongoing assessment and series of rearrangements necessary to support the growth of the human styled species.

In total there have been six major restarts or alterations of the human race spanning a period of the last two to three million years. The Sataan energy is drawn from strains of rainbow energy emanating into the Ancient arena. It uses the Cosmos Proper as a base to further the exploratory work assigned through the direction of those responsible for invoking the Divine Plan. The strains of rainbow energy are cosmic and not confined to complementing any one persona or family.

Important levels of self-discovery were opened for the Ancients by dropping planet Earth and certain creatures now known as humans into the atmospheric density described as the third dimension. What is density and what is the cause of memory loss? We call it the sea of forgetfulness. It is an area of darkness within the depths of fluidity that are defined by atmospheric pressures.

The messages of human movement and further development were recorded in the memory brain as coded symbols in the psyche. The translation of the symbols into activity is the role of the individual mind. Dirty or grubby minds usually mean there is transference of misinformation. There has been and still is in many cases much superstitious interference in the human mind because of deep seated flaws that built a wall of dogma from religious fears. We call this cause god sense that overloads the systems in the human ego with the arrogance of superior judgement.

That Sataan energy is a major influence on human behaviour is affirmed. However, the Christian religious pundits snarled their lines when they declared Lucifer and the devil were part of the same entity as Satan. Each is a different entity, forming from different strains of greater energy and work from different levels. 20 years ago the Devil entity was obliged to leave the planet and we are given to understand has reverted into harmless energy.

Within ourselves we have no interest in the goo of planetary worship called religion. The idea of Almighty God was introduced as an iconic pattern to comfort the mindless human sheep needing bell-wethers called prophets, monks, ministers and priests, whatever, to give aberrated counsel and extract their asking price accordingly. Nor do we much care about the vagaries of human superstitions as such except to give an overview of some of the early beginnings in mythology when requested.

Because religious controls have been imposed from elsewhere in the cosmos they are a foreign interference operating without basic foundation. Religious people will say their input of energy in society comes from love as all things do. However, their credos have been built from a base of subliminal fears and the necessity for maintaining controls over the fears of others is paramount in their teachings.

So the many stories from past events are to be revealed and the beliefs fed to people will crumble and tumble as the eyes of the world witnessed the implosion of the twin towers, the event of 911, which heralded the pending collapse of super powers and the tyranny that prospered by the controllers of corruption.

Among many areas of disclosure will be the demise of religions because the practice of idolistic worship, fashioned and adorned by the ego support of god sense, is reaching the end of its days. The lies that have built the empires of religious deceit are to be made clear to fully open the eyes of half-awake planetary children.

Today on planet Earth there are mixes of cosmic entities representing a variety of greater energy sources existing beyond the cosmos. These intrepid volunteers are nominated as cosmic pioneers who have entered once more onto the planet in recent times to do the bidding of the Great Mother. One reason is to draw the curtain on the involvement of external influences determining the lives and loves of humans in the third dimension. The purpose is to effectively declare a prearranged cosmic birthing enabling planet Earth and its habitat creatures a re-entry into the cosmic arena that their original ancestors left so abruptly many eons ago.

Initial Birthing of Planet Earth

Many million years ago were it to be measured in planetary time a conference of interesting and interested entities representing various areas of cosmic energy took place in the great meeting hall of Ancients situated in the Cosmos Proper.

The discussion was centred on the recent building of planet Earth, and its future purpose, which in most eyes was undetermined because of a lack of proportional information. The occasion took place before third dimensional linear time and space as humans are conditioned to wear came on line. Such empirical measurements if acknowledged then were mentally subjective and only relative to sequential movements.

Who was to be responsible for the shaping of its future life events now the planet was functioning was the open question on the table for debate. What was even more pressing was the issue of mankind, delineated so far as they understood to be a specified creature of form independent of nature.

Without the availability of a delivered program, a blueprint from the resources of an undetermined greater energy field, creative materials were becoming diminished. Therefore, leftovers from other planetary building systems were being brought out and dusted off. Then they were utilized haphazardly in a manner of sticking together a framework of sorts into the proposed being called man. It was somewhat like building a cosmic scarecrow with odd scraps of extra bits and pieces. Was there to be any genuine purpose involved in the exercise at hand? That question was fast becoming a bone of contention.

Somehow the patchwork differences in human colouring had developed into a splitting of unified patterns within the cosmic order of the entity/energies. The design from the diamond template was for some incomprehensible reason becoming separated into half-shapes of dualistic type pyramids.

There was concern, even consternation, from those whose prescient vision saw limitations being imposed on any progressive development. Then there were others who argued that opposing factors would productively build friction and in turn futuristic ventures could be power driven by such excessive heat to return gainful dividends working effectively in their favour.

In this manner imposing factions on a cosmic level set patterns for a future human submersion into the duality of mind. 'You cannot name to us one thing that is an opposite,' said the nature elementals to the Ancients, putting a case for proliferating abundance en masse without separation.

The Ancients of the Father pedigree gave consideration to what was being stated. 'You are right,' they agreed, 'as far as your areas are concerned. But hu-man (emphasizing the duality split) creatures are not being made to be natural so your vision does not encompass them. We have installed a series of mind programs, as extended principles from The One, for the purpose of cosmic experiment.

So settle back and watch our creation in play as the games of Olympus unfold, as the survival techniques of planetary causes go head to head with the universal in-laws of fellow planets. The conditioning of brute force survival tactics versus the intellect of guided worship will be displayed. Powerful actions shall be demonstrated and played out in formations of dual purpose. What a masterpiece in living cosmic colour is to be enacted.'

As the words were spoken a leader of the Ancients held aloft the shining sword of Intelligence, in which the energy field glowed brightly with the light of will and power.

The Line of Mothers then present conferred and shook their heads, resolutely combined in their decision, and with one voice decreed. 'If that is the game devised for the human species then you will play it out without the support of female energy. Wisdom and beauty, which was to be our major contribution in kindness, will never take sides with acts of cruelty. We have instructed the Angels to remove our cosmic essence from the games. Therefore the unrestricted flow of Love energy is no longer made available.'

Swift as an arrow at a signal from the Divine Mother, designated to be the world nurturer, the hand of Sataan snatched away the upheld sword on display and in one swift and sure movement drove it into the capstone of human destiny, which effectively removed the availability of cosmic memory.

Once more the Divine Mother spoke: 'Let the sword remain so buried until one shall come onto the planet with the strength of cosmic understanding to heal the pain of mental division between presence and essence. Hitherto the light of Love energy in cosmic glow will only be shown on planet Earth by reflection. Intelligence of a greater order shall remain hidden from the sight of humankind until the sword is drawn out from the stone through a divine family agreement'.

As a gesture of further denial the Divine Mother veiled her features and the Angels drew a line across the planetary face of Earth, thus determining that the full light of consciousness would split between darkness and light of day, with shadows daily cast to invoke purpose in seeking unresolved memories.

Some of the Ancients laughed uproariously and one called Yahweh spoke forth in full arrogance born of male ignorance: 'How like a woman. When was there ever gain without some pain involved? We will match your curse with curse. Let the women of planet Earth then bear their children in pain. Let them pay homage to men as their masters, as their keepers. Let all women forever forget their allegiance sworn to this Great Mother mystery.'

Lightning flashed from the internal eye of the Dark Mother who had remained silent until then. 'The cosmic colourings are denied from the games so there will be no completion. We are removing two of the seven rings until the Great Mother energy be recognised and restored into human memory.'

Some of the Ancient ones roared with rage at what they saw as impertinence of the female energy. Once more Yahweh spoke with tones of lurid vehemence. 'Then let your dark blood flow as a monthly reminder that planetary women are to be seen as the weaker sex and female values do not and cannot match the level of male standards'.

The women withdrew their presence, leaving the line of Fathers to further the Ancient cause off course. As the games began the criss-crossing lines of figuration emphasizing confrontation were to be indelibly marked into the psyche of Earth people like some gigantic fireworks display of noughts and crosses. The greater intelligence representing The One stepped even further back allowing the human psyche to formulate a series of various playing fields of subterfuge; where the human mind, unfortunately, found each level strewn with self sabotaging measures that relentlessly destroyed superior type civilizations of their varied makings.

The Angels lit candles for a remembrance of human purpose and the future destiny of planet Earth becoming a showpiece visible in the cosmic fields became a lost cause. Meanwhile the reflected lantern light of planetary knowledge bestowed a mentally arrogant attitude born from a partitioned Ancient ignorance, which defiantly entered yet another biased form sheet lacking suitable balance and support into the surface memory banks of the people inhabiting planet Earth.

The male generated power of a surface ego management continues to this day, insisting that what matters most is what people are, or becoming, and survival of systematic controls is all that counts. The daily emphasis is still given to the ego mind as lauded knowledge remains on lantern power and has to work overtime to maintain self-esteem as a teetering framework upholding misguided patterns of belief.

Sadly, what has resulted from these unbalanced projections of loaded esteem is a recipe for humans receiving even more painful global events, which offers even less accountability to endorsing that which is deemed worthwhile in the progressive development of a greater cosmic understanding.

The Hidden Wells of Life

One day in some forgettable spread
Thereof by chance an article read
Written by some regrettable authority
Whose immature mind made decree
On weighty matters of significant post
Bemoaning the fact that life was lost
There being no longer any physical haste
To conquer horizons, nor lands to waste

I laughed with some strange knowing
That if he were correct in his showing
Then man is compelled beyond rescue
To turn inward where self is on review

Tainted wells of hellish fire dwell there
In causes lost from lives spent in prayer
While emotion waves vary in belied state
In psychic forests where wild beasts wait

For those with courage prepared to task
Mental blocks of the many afraid to ask
One lesser step therein strains to repair
Till nothingness drains minds of dull despair

Chapter III.

Angels

Walking and Talking in Harmony with Angels

Angels can be described as sparks of light energy operating throughout the cosmos on behalf of greater energy beings who have more than a working interest in human advancement. Let us state clearly that we are not an authority on Angels or their perceived overview of happenings as they occur. We act as willing conduits with those beings of light energy who convey to us specific information regarding the realization of greater understanding and the imminent rearrangement of human affairs on planet Earth.

Operating beyond the mental barriers of ego controlled thinking is any amount of multiple entity/energies moving throughout planetary life and their extensive reach of agreement goes well beyond the cosmic movement in which humans are soon to be involved. The numbers are comprised of Angels, Star People, Ancients representing as Father energy, a Line of Mothers, Greater energy, plus untold other players who have had a say in playing past events and many that are still active in the future advancement of human endeavour.

There are countless levels of featured existence in the Cosmos; namely areas occupied by those who are in receipt of Angel direction, influencing the drift of planetary life through the elective use of divine intelligence.

Though for people presently situated as Earth inhabitants having any understanding of Angel movement and the areas of their integrated and purposeful work is well outside the range of average human comprehension. These beings of light work in realms beyond the limitations of ego related ideas and ideals, in which controlling mindsets are still binding and blinding planetary people within their constrained areas by a locked down number of sensory patterns requiring release.

Are Angels real? Angels are part of certain existences that are recognisable to those not bound hand and foot by the ignorance and arrogance of mental conditioning. Children do not have to understand Angels. To small children Angels and also fairies and other elemental creatures are instinctively part of their early childhood existence.

Angels have no interest in listening or taking sides in human arguments.

As stated Angels are beings of light without physical bodies that carry any amount of form acknowledged in times immemorial. They are part of energy resonances that operate at different degrees or levels throughout various cosmic fields. The various levels are difficult to explain in planetary terms. To the human mind levels can appear as horizontal lines stretching between benchmarks. In angelic terms levels are degrees of cosmic interaction working impressively towards expansion. When we wish to mentally explore beyond the third dimensional limits into cosmic levels it is only possible to move there without the aid of scientifically given references that are empirically misconstrued.

Angels do not disappear because scientific instruments cannot measure them.

Scientists deny the unexplainable and extraneous occurrences that have been recorded throughout eons of previous times by labelling metaphysical activity as unworldly. What that simply means both mentally and physically there is activity beyond the scope of their minds and limited instruments to record and analyse phenomena beyond the enclosed barriers imposed by scientific rules of engagement. As such they insist that mysteries or what is evidenced beyond their limited understanding should be declared as unrealistic and dismissed as fantasy.

So there is much to be revealed and monitored when we escape the restricted confines of a planetary trapped third dimensional existence. Soon all that religious orders hold sacrosanct, along with esoteric man's so-called security reliance on scientific jargon, are doomed to tumble and crumble before being rearranged and rebuilt.

The pain of separation, emanating from the human system as it does regularly in a constant emotional exhaust of fear, drives the urges of excess in societal beliefs today. Such inhibiting fear factors that are lacking in vital formats of energy will soon enough leak to the surface of the rational mind and when they become obvious will be summarily surrendered or dismissed.

Humanity will learn to reject the lures of excitable habit along with its convenient memory lapses of forgetting past errors of judgement. Certain people when given fresh information will start to awaken anew and remember who they are, where they have come from, and what future benefits their purposeful roles on the planet are bound to display.

In this newfound vision of life, advisedly named the dawning of a New Day, the Angels will play any number of appropriate roles in offering human guidance. As will the cosmic players dressed in human form that have been deliberately scattered around the planet to assist in awakening ordinary people into realizing a new found fifth dimensional experience.

Do not believe in Angels. Beliefs set in the mind of humans are like tacky hanging paper that smells sweet and attracts flies. Angels do not require or request anyone to believe in them. Instead, give over outworn ideas on birthing and dying of planetary life being temporal. Such old style types of religious led thinking have had their use by date.

See the beliefs you were trained into endorsing as a child, and most still carry, as no more than conditioned balloons filled with hot air, which they always were. Release your mental attachment to them and watch them float away into empty space. Where humankind is shortly destined to go there is no space reserved for beliefs. They are just extra baggage, like the weight of emotional drag, which when retained in memory only weighs the ignorant and arrogant minds of superior type people further down.

There is a new level of post-scientific information soon to be made available, which will show clearly that the memory of past experiences is no longer a necessary recall to precede a new world order of greater understanding nominated cosmically as the Fifth Dimension. What will become obvious is that the human endeavour to climb, described as evolution, has always been preceded by a greater order of divine planning.

When the belief in duality, the common error promoting freewill and choice on this planet, falls over the Angels will be standing and applauding. So will those presently in human bodies who heed the timely advisement on offer from the Angels. Their planetary role is to prepare themselves adequately for the oncoming cosmic events that will rearrange the unseemly conscious patterns governing everyday life.

Observation

How do Angels communicate with us? Through various methods of channelling, such as deliberate signage posted along the way, and fresh thoughts coming into our heads, which we call left field advisement. Angels listen in on our conversations and are not backward in coming forward to explain whenever our interpretations have gone wayward.

The Angels advise us that Love as the core of living energy is on its way. It has not arrived fully as yet though it can be felt momentarily as vibration. That is until the foggy areas of the mind and the melting ice around the heart settle back into imbalanced positioning again. The upsetting circumstances of the present world scenes are pictographs of humans experiencing the winter chills of bitter desperation before the New Day comes celebrating a springtime that is duly arriving post haste.

The dawning of realization for the people of their cosmic inheritance is coming ever closer to fruition. The veil covering the face of the Divine Mother has been lifted since late 1996 and the New Day is sending in the first rays of a deeper comprehension portraying an advancement of Life and Living Free. The people of planet Earth are being awakened gradually to realize their cosmic inheritance. The cosmic Angels stand ever ready to guide the lost children Home on behalf of the Great Mother.

The Messenger

13th August 2022

The dishes of another Saturday dinner are quickly cleared away as Jézel suddenly feels the familiar pressure building in her head. We repair with reasonable haste to the lounge room, the seat of the Hollow Arena.

Messenger: Well, good evening.

Unnamed: Hello.

Aria: Good evening.

Messenger: The light is dimming on planet Earth, but it is a false light that is dimming; a false light built on a false premise. It is bringing much fear, concern, waves of hatred, waves of doubt, and let us say clearly, we are still on this planet depthing. So there is still a movement into the nadir. You who are pioneers on the other hand have to come out of the nadir and move into the spiral towards the light. So you have to do a quick step. Know how to dance...quickstep?

Know that the planet and its people are moving inexorably into the Fifth Dimension. Know that you are shining lights to direct people to a greater understanding. Know that there are others of your ilk that are still lost and wandering, wondering, and that you are to let them know. You are to give direction. But not without realizing, giving them the understanding of the enormity.

You are not giving them freebies. This is not some game where you say, 'we are love and light and we will let you pass through, no matter how you want to do it, or whatever you want to do'. There is a procedure. As much as you are not in it for gain you are to partake in an exchange. They are not going to climb on your coattails without that exchange. Let us be very clear. There is a procedure.

And yes, of course it is to be done through agreement. Because these are shifting times and everybody is in it for a buck or two, for what they can get. There are a lot of false people, false in wanting gain for themselves without having the agreement and the balance with others. Greed, selfishness in that respect will not work. Do not be beguiled by those who are out to get what they can without an exchange.

So each day you inch closer to being more prominent and being more obvious. So each and every day you are to be more aware of the enormity of the undertaking...we have used that word twice now...and also the importance of ever working with harmlessness; having no interest in outcomes or even incomes. We are going to be making sure that these will even out. It hasn't happened yet but we are working for that to occur.

Again, these dark times on planet Earth are not going to improve any time soon. Not because that is the way we want it. We are looking at planet Earth and its people plummeting as far as possible before it is able to regain ground and have the allowance to move into dimension that allows people to move freely. Okay, that is a small look. It is not the fullness. Needless to say, there is much more to be opened up in this new

Awakening to a New Mind

level that we are approaching. Let's say that we are approaching; let us not say that the Fifth Dimension is coming to us. Let's say we, and it is all inclusive, are approaching the Fifth Dimension. It can all be in the perspective in this time in the history of planet Earth and its people.

You are no small fry. You may be sitting in the back blocks and not be noticed by all and sundry. You may be passed by, by 99.99% of people on planet Earth, but we are with you a hundred percent. You are our grounding area, from where our work can proceed. And we thank you.

In unison the Unnamed and Aria say, 'We thank you too'.

Messenger: Good evening to you.

Chapter IV.

The Divine Family

1980

Veil of the Mother

*Black rocks, sand bathed
In a moonlit glow
Where a woman walks serene
One shoulder bare
Yet she did wear
The raiment of a queen*

*She walks with me
Yet does not speak
Her face is hidden
Where I cannot see
So I must seek
Her constantly
Past life or love forbidden?*

Luxor: This poem is drawn from a waking dream that I experienced some 40 odd years ago. The setting seemed to me like the shores of the

Aegean Sea, an area I have not visited in this lifetime. I was seated on the sand some 20 metres from the water and watched while she bathed her feet in the sudsy foam. The Lady was dark haired and purposeful in her movements while serenity was etched in every graceful line of her form. It was 16 more years before she revealed her presence as the Divine Mother.

Arrival on Earth - The Divine Family

Entering the Cosmos Proper

The cosmic centre where the capsule carrying the **Divine Family** of four entity/energies landed millions of years ago is like a large metropolis we reference as the Cosmos Proper. The Cosmos Proper was well and truly set in place before the solar systems that surround the Shining Ones referenced as stars appeared. It is a central area of cosmic work very similar to a New York typesetting that opens up different enterprises and places them out into the rest of the world for the purpose of expanded development. It is a cosmic hub of progressive development, if you like, working assiduously throughout the astral fields.

Cosmic Players you have met in the second and third Chapters

The Cosmos Proper is situated in no specific dimension, has no time span that human minds can comprehend, and no identifiable space available for scientific measurement. It is inhabited by a male order of talented players we call Ancients and a female line of Mothers. There are Angels present in their varied orders of cosmic duty, and Elementals as builders, nurturers and carers of nature projects are also represented. The Angels though they have come from beyond the Cosmos inhabit the various arenas for the benefit of assisting those required to develop fresh areas of cosmic design.

Veil of Separation

Traces of such timeless existence are still retained though contained within the distant memories of the human psyches. This planetary area of modern times called Earth has been enclosed by a veil of separation causing a breakdown in regulated galactic communications for millions of years measured in linear time. So it is beyond the capacity of average mental thought processing in the minds of humans to easily accept and realize the grandeur of distanced cosmic relations.

Sea of Forgetfulness & Love

The rational minds of humans are set at its present levels of limitation by third dimensional depthing. The minds of regulated people are enclosed within vacant bubbles in a sea of forgetfulness commonly referenced as atmosphere. Therefore people cannot comprehend the cosmic arenas we are commissioned to speak of by using normal thought processing that relies on the accuracy of planetary memory. However, be assured Love is energy that bonds within all things, is beyond all things and promotes and embraces life whether it is understandable or no in any given moment.

Let us just reiterate the confounding history of planet Earth and its people. It is one mighty recount and worthy of retelling from a different perspective.

Earth into the third dimension & Solar System

Two and half million linear years ago Earth and its incubated creatures referenced initially as Man was moved from its nursery status and located into this solar system we call the Universe and then was sunk to an atmospheric level science names as the third dimension. Part of our recovery work in memory is to realign the distorted stories that have been fed to people through the self-proclaimed authorities registered as societies, which are namely answerable for endorsing the inaccurate beliefs of both religion and science.

Introducing Jésu and Lucifer

The Ancients play the roles of architectural designers of planets, builders of enterprises of the same, as well they have a responsibility to maintain contact and provide updates and upkeep of the innumerable planets that they have set into motion. There are more Ancients than is possible for human minds to assess, but our planetary interest is focussed in recounting the stories of Lucifer and Jésu, the twin sons of the Divine Family, and by extension their association with humans on planet Earth is directed towards the wishes of the Divine Mother and one who agreeably answers to the name of Sataan.

Grandeur of Cosmic Family

This planetary area occupied by humanity has been enclosed by a veil put in place more than two million years ago causing a serious breakdown in advancing galactic communications. So it is beyond the average capacity of human thought to realize the grandeur of their cosmic families operating outside the solar system.

Explanation of Planet Earth into Solar System

At the request of the Divine Mother the final stages of planet Earth were built in the cosmos proper under the instruction of Sataan. Like a wandering small child, Earth was enticed to move too close to a dividing fence line and got sucked into this solar system where it began its fixed orbit from the depths of the third dimension. Later at the further behest of the Divine Mother planet Venus was built as a sister energy and entered into this solar system as a companion aligning with Earth. Venus is known cosmically as the planet of love.

Venus

However, Venus was not sucked in. It was deliberately placed into its orbital position it still occupies. When Venus came into its set program it smashed apart a makeshift planet that was already lodged in its designated orbital space. That planet was like what the Ancients would refer to as a low-level dilapidated energy, so it was of no great consequence to break it up. Like builders today would have no problem in demolishing a tired building on an old site, by razing the area and breaking up the old concrete base to replace it with a new structuring.

The energy of the Divine Family is firmly seated in planet Earth today and working to make its presence and essence known and felt. This world of people is soon to be awakened from its slumberous mode to recall its cosmic birthright and future purpose as both mind and brain becomes unshackled from relying on stories of an unremembered past.

The Divine Family prior to the Birthing of Planet Earth: The Introduction of Living Fire

The light ran throughout the cosmos like a series of blue veins. It was a blue lightning, which fed from itself and drew fresh patterns from its own energy field. When it reached a designated spot it paused and from the hollowed vein an egg was deposited.

These blue veins or energy rays of light emanated throughout the void of darkness thus causing the birthing of new life wherever the consigned eggs were deposited. The particular one that is of interest to humans was delivered into the Cosmos Proper through the efforts of the Shining Ones and was nurtured by Angels long before Earth was built and linear time began registration. It came with four strands of energy in an egg type capsule that merged for the journey a particular strain known cosmically as the Divine Family.

Deference is not usually a feature of cosmic energy because of the inherent understandings of **Truth, Equality**, and **Unity**. However, the angelic energies were aware that they were witnessing a beginning of something special. The Divine Family as presented carried an aura of beauty and strength that was a remembering for those that were privy to the arrival. The family, acknowledged as divine because of its energy, was welcomed into the extended family of cosmic workers performing in the Cosmos Proper.

When the Angels opened the delivered egg as it arrived in the Cosmos Proper there were four entity/energies enclosed within. There was the Father. There was the Mother. There were two nominated as sons who appeared in the form of babes. The sons were joined at the hip in the sense of what humans would describe as Siamese twins. The Angels separated them. The names of the Divine Family that were taken on are titles and are to be seen as symbolic. The Father and the Mother are not parents of the two sons. Not in the sense that the human mind could understand as parenting. The four entity/energies represented varied areas of interest that extended far beyond the cosmic realms.

The Divine Family in its merged context represented a royal Blue Bloodline

The energy of the Family carries strains of divinity far beyond any planetary ideas of godship and worship. Nor can they be termed as sexual in bodies formed beyond the cosmos. They carry the blue blood of those known cosmically as royals, which is a royal blue that comes from realms beyond the cosmic fields.

They are acknowledged as entities from a greater energy field that is able to produce their personalities into regions of interest. It is not that the energy in itself carries personalities as such. Energy in action displays vibrancies of sound and colour. When they move into a dimension for the purpose of working in the area they are required to adopt a persona.

The different roles of the energies emerged as father, mother and twin sons or suns, known as Jésu and Lucifer.

The Mother shares the light of beauty and wisdom that can be expressed through female energy. The Father provided the male energy portraying will and drive. Jésu carries Truth formed through the strain of Christos Energy. Lucifer, known also as the 'Unnamed One', carries the cosmic torch of Intelligence that offers to people advanced consciousness levels of greater understanding. These are gifts for human progression and can be bestowed upon those on the planet who make themselves available in service to the Great Mother and thus deemed worthy. *The family is symbolic for the purpose of guidance in the advancement of human endeavour.*

The two sons enjoyed the benefits flowing from these adult energies. They were placed in the care of Angels and when they grew of a suitable age they were inducted into the teaching of the Ancients. Then they were put to work in the cosmic fields amongst star energies, areas overviewed by Ancients, Angels and Elementals. That is a brief background to their arrival in the cosmos.

The Disagreement

Our story then moves across to a small planet that was being nurtured in the Cosmos Proper nursery. The planet in its future third dimensional position would become known as Earth. For the time being the creatures on the planet, among them those known as a species called Man, slept peacefully in the prepared womb of the Great Mother.

'As above, so below' holds significant meaning for those who are prepared to sit still, wait patiently and listen intently. So it is necessary to see that a planet in its early making was similar to a small child. In the cosmic field it is nurtured by energies that maintain and surround it. So the planet Earth was created from the efforts of Greater Energy at the behest of the Divine Mother, which means it was born into the Cosmos. In that early stage it achieved a sense of consciousness and inevitably became a toddler. Then it was assigned to the care of one of the Sons whose energy has been recorded on planet Earth in different times as Baal and Jesus.

One day as stories tend to unfold the little planet strayed too close to its cosmic limit and was sucked into an outer area known today as the universal solar system rotating around the star energy named as Ra. This turn of an unexplained event started a disagreement between the members of the Divine family. One brother, known through that period of time as Lucifer, having observed the difficulty and pain being suffered by the forsaken creatures was determined that the planet and creatures should be returned to its cosmic nursery.

He was able by over viewing methods to see the dire straits of the creatures as they struggled to come to terms with the shock of their new surroundings located in the third dimension. In particular the creatures named as man were prostrate, bellies down flat on the ground, wriggling like worms when they were initially designed to walk upright in the manner of cosmic people.

He made his opinion known loud and clear that someone in authority had well and truly made a huge mistake that needed rectifying to those who were prepared to listen. The Father did not agree with his viewpoint. The Father was of the opinion that there were greater energies at work than they were aware of and that the family would do best to sit and wait for future outcomes to be revealed. The discussions in the divine family soon became heated disagreements.

Lucifer was young and headstrong. The Father was adamant. Eventually the Mother was drawn in and she also argued with the Father's opinion. They were not happy times. Until then the Divine Family had been a model of unity. The four members were now distracted, distanced and distraught. There were no signs of a ready resolution. There never is while in the throes of heated argument.

Question Time at the Table

The Story of Lucifer backing Human Suffrage

Prelude to the Divine Family Argument

Lucifer has been absent from the Cosmos Proper for some time on star runner duties and was unaware of the removal of the man species from its incubation period on to planet Earth. From the viewing platform he is horrified to see the tiny creatures crawling around on their bellies in reptilian fashion.

Questioning

He realizes that their opportunity to sustain life is fraught with danger and loses no time in questioning his family as to what measures are being taken to rectify the situation. Lucifer faces the Divine Father across the table where the Divine Mother and Jésu are also sharing the evening meal. He is angry at the noncommittal responses he receives and is determined to get a result from his line of questioning.

'I want to know why Earth and its creatures are still not seated in the crèche position. Who ordered its removal? Who dropped it into that atmospheric hellhole, the Angels are calling the third dimension? The species called Man cannot stand. They are crawling on their stomachs like reptiles. They were not built with the stabilizing strength of reptilian energy. They cannot survive if they remain in that state for any period of time.'

The Father pushes back from the table and meets Lucifer's gaze with one equally as strong.

'Who are you to question those who call the shots on when and where life on each planet goes? I do not know who ordered it, but I do know to stay out of areas that are not my concern. You would do well to do the same.'

'I cannot and I will not', comes the rapid reply. 'I was not raised to ignore the cries of creatures in distress. I did not take the vow of equality to walk away from pain because it is deemed by some to not be in my area.' He turns and appeals to Jésu. 'They are people designated to be in your care. Into your hands was given the guardianship of the planet and its creatures. You were given responsibility. How can you take what is happening so lightly?'

Jésu straightens his frame and gives Lucifer a searching look. He recognizes the signs of distress in his brother and that he is close to tears. He also knows from past experience that when Lucifer appears vulnerable it is then that the Great Dragon energy he carries is most likely to surge through his system, causing him to apply massive pressure on those who appear to oppose him.

'Steady, brother, I do not take it lightly. All the information is not available yet so how can we have a full understanding of the event or occasion? When the time is right we will be advised what to do.'

The response from Lucifer is heated. 'In the meantime they suffer. They are children that call out for their father and what I see and hear is indifference to their plight. It is enough said. If I cannot get a hearing here I know those who are more prepared to understand and remedy these pathetic circumstances.'

The Father is stung by the suggestion he is uncaring. 'I will tell it to you one more time; stay out of that area. Your bullheadedness will only make matters worse.'

Lucifer turns to the Divine Mother for understanding. She puts a finger to his lips. 'Enough has been said for now,' and her words of wise counsel are law to Lucifer. 'Come and speak with me when your head is cooler and clearer.'

Lucifer stands up, hesitates as though there is more he would like to say, and then strides out of the room. The three remaining members of the Divine Family sit for a short while until the Father breaks the silence. 'I never could handle his petulance. Why cannot he ever see that some worlds are being built many times over as prototypes, to be experimental, used for that purpose solely and then dismantled?'

The Divine Mother's words come soft and firm. 'That is not the case with the people of planet Earth. Lucifer may at times appear hasty. He comes from a flow of energy that invariably at times seems to be at odds with others, yet events have shown he has an instinct for touching base with what is appropriate."

The Father throws a look of scorn. 'Spoken like a devoted mother. He was a contrary child who was allowed to play too long with fairies. He was doted on by foster Angels and tutored by an outcast from the Ancient inner circle. Yes, he has a way with him when it comes to working order into cosmic fields, but look at those he hangs around with. The likes of Charlie. What is his cover?

All we ever hear from him are exploits of barroom brawling. Some kind of example to the students we are training in the Ancient corp. And that battle cry or song or whatever it is of 'All for One and One for all'. Yes, I know we serve the One, but they throw it around as though they are the ones that are being given preference.'

A smile lights the Mother's face. 'They are young and carefree. Duty will sober them soon enough. In the meantime let us not use our mealtimes for argument.' Jésu rises, kisses the Mother on the cheek, gives a high five to the Father and leaves.

The Father goes to speak, considers for a moment, and then leaves for a meeting with the Ancients. The Mother sits for a moment as in a dream state and then softly claps her hands. An attendant Angel steps into the room. 'Have a courier convey to Sataan that I wish a private audience'.

****

Lucifer sought the advice of a certain mentor known for his ability to make things happen in an orderly fashion. He advised that if Lucifer was resolved to gain the return of the planet then he was prepared to assist. The events that followed that discussion have had a marked impact and effect on the conditioning of the planet and on the development of all entity/energies concerned.

The Landing of the 37

The Song of 37

Listen to the stories
The Angels like to tell
Of the call to courage
When the 37 fell

Diving in deep waters
Where man was not complete
The daring 37
Put humans on their feet

Now other times are over
The marquees coming down
Ring the bell of changes
The circus leaves the town

The acting has been ended
The players take their bow
The thorn of pain suspended
Upon Love's golden bough

Chorus
How many times it's happened
Far too many to repeat
Each return of 37
Puts humans on their feet

In a planned elliptical formation we, referenced in the cosmic records as the 37, a small group of cosmic pioneers, dropped down into this electromagnetic bubble called the third dimension and landed on planet Earth two and a half million years ago. Periodically, we return to the planet in the guise of human form to assist the forward progression of people reaching for their purposeful goals. This time we have successfully grounded a working post, called the Hollow Arena, enabling a flow of regular communication with beyond cosmic advocates who intentionally sent us forth to repair the broken strands separating humans from their cosmic origins.

Recently, we have rounded the extended base of our journey in a looping style and have only just begun to climb the incline to hasten our journey homewards. There are still many tie offs ahead for us before we can fully reclaim our birthright, along with those of the planetary people, whose destiny though nominated in the divine plan, falls short of cosmic energy, which is not yet available for general use on planet Earth.

What can be said though in regard to the eagle exchanges and also with the serpent energy is that we have been instrumental in breaking the back of a cosmic puzzle we were initially presented with in scattered form. Though what happened to the 37 then may seem like eons ago in distance measured by time and space, that birthing episode was not accurately described as it appeared then, nor has it been suitably presented to half-crazed people on planet Earth obsessed or possessed with third dimensional credulity that is hopelessly out of balance.

Some modern scientists have called their minimal endeavours in space travel cognition as reaching for the stars, but for those of us who were cosmic star runners when planet Earth was still in the design stages we are awakened in memory to know we are under direction to complete what is to be part of the final loop in a set progressive movement of future cosmic development. Effectively, with the advent of the Fifth Dimension hovering overhead we are moving into the early processes of straightening our course for our cosmic home.

As cosmic pioneers breaking open new ground or territory we are here to share our conveyed learning with those people on planet Earth willing to advance beyond the present day mental restrictions of duality and polarity.

For the past 25 years cast as players in human form we have been engaged in digging and diving into locked down regions of the psyche with the specific interest of uncovering the nominated hidden pearls beyond price. This requires a disclosure within cosmic memory to advance a greater understanding of human existence, thus realizing our dedicated involvement in progressing the wares of Love and Intelligence.

What wonderful world recordings held within the silent psyche vaults are soon to be recognized, acknowledged, and made available for use in developing fresh stages of comprehensive activity, firstly to rearrange the present day human mental design, which will assist in realigning cosmic relativity in the longer term.

What mysteries can be further unravelled as people apply genius styles of research into probing the living formations of star systems whose records are retained in files beyond cosmic memory. In the utilisation of these submerged patterns when unfolded people will be competent to draw on essential information to be accepting of New Life programs and a Living Free arrangement in mind delivered from available quarters, a mystifying arena, that which has been termed by some as no-time and no-space, which we nominate as nothingness.

****

Two and a half million years ago the face of the Divine Mother was veiled. The energy of the Father line then became paramount and was reflected onto planet Earth. The will and drive portrayed through the Father energy was converted into male power because it well suited the density mix in the third dimension.

Present Day Events of the Divine Family - 2006

The Divine Family has progressively merged to where the Mother and Father are acknowledged as one. The Father has converged within the Mother energy. It is time for the human family to become aware of past circumstances and meet with the Divine Mother. The separation that denies humanity the memory of its birthright has been in place two and a half million years. Yet when the psyche memory clicks in, like a computer setting, the recall of past events is instant.

Since the veil has been removed from the Divine Mother's face can people on the planet begin to remember her smile, her warmth, and her open arms offering a tender embrace? The grace, the beauty, and charm are available to those who take her hand and learn there are simple ways of settling differences without the abuse of harmful destruction.

She is the bearer of wisdom and beauty, style and grace. She calls now to her Earth children to put down their tools of advantage. To lay aside their futile tantrums of rage that only do damage unto their selves. It is time for her distraught and tormented children to rest. Will you speak openly with her? She is waiting to hear your voice. If you lift your head and listen you will hear her call. It is a call being made to each and every one of her lost children to return Home.

****

As stated earlier the Divine family has two sons. They are twins. Wherever one appears on the planet Earth in the flesh the other one invariably supports behind the scenes. Now in these times they will appear together as Jésu and Lucifer without the masks they oft times previously wore.

To assist in the transition of people from the third dimension to the fifth dimension the two sons, Jésu and Lucifer, working on behalf of the Divine Mother, are presently engaged in human form on planet Earth. It is their role with the assistance of some other team members to anchor the energy of LOVE into the planet. They are assisting in making the awakening transition period from the third to the fifth dimension as smooth a venture as possible for the Earth bound creatures being required to make the shift.

The species of man who moved into the formation of human beings when they first experienced the light of consciousness and found their feet are to become party to the unification with divine energy. It is a divinity without the imposed limitations of god worship. Humans are destined to join in a stream of Life fashioned through the energy of Love and bring unto each a combined understanding of their cosmic heritage. The energy that flows from sharing with the family is to become their strength. What divisive force, being locked down in planetary effort, can withstand the energy flow of Love that is administered from the Divine Plan?

The planetary slates of divisive male control are being wiped clean. In the awareness of a New Day where humans are fast approaching there awaits their cosmic destiny. There is a new energy growth in living whole and free, designed to restore Love and joy, which arrives through the welcoming embrace of the Divine Family.

Coming home is to embrace your cosmic family. The Divine Mother waits with open arms. Let go of the ego confinement of mind and memory to come home to ME.

****

Members of the Divine Family

The symbolic emblems the family carries are nominated as the Diamond, the Rose, the Cross, and the Star. The star can also be signified as a down-turned sword and is synonymous with the cross. The four combine to carry the basic colours of the rainbow. The diamond relates to yellow, the rose is green, the cross is red and the star is blue.

The Divine energy projected and manifested is displayed as part of a constellation visible in the night sky as the Southern Cross. Four of the five stars are representative of the Divine Family. Would it come as a surprise for people to liken Jésu to star energy? Every human carries a portion of one star or another. If they could only fix their eyes upon that denotable star they could walk off this planet and not be required to return without their agreement.

Divine Mother and Introducing Divine Womanhood
May 2010

Divine Mother: I come not here to give you answers. There is a part inside you that is me and that is you. Love is the essence. It is within and without. Around and about. Above and below. It distils the wine we call Angel juice. It is available to those who give themselves over. Till now it has lain dormant within the wellsprings of humans. Now it is time for the awakening.

****

The significance of what we are to say is not to be specifically directed to a relay of any one person, though it is the Divine Mother energy that registers the early lead in Womanhood. It is SHE who offers the wisdom and beauty for those who will represent Divine Womanhood and others similar in kind who will carry understandings that are so important to be heard, absorbed and thus clearly understood by those with ears to listen.

The Divine Mother is the producer of this present day shift in energy, which welcomes in the New Day. She is asking her lost children to remember who they are and make the commitment to come Home. The chaos, both planetary and humanistic, which is occurring at present on the global stage is partly being caused by emotional traumas resurfacing from the distant past. When we agreeably allow ourselves to hold the hand of the Mother she assists us in clearing away the backlog of unresolved issues.

For two and a half million years the family was split by disagreement. Not anymore. Nearly 26 years ago on the tenth day of November 1996 a ceremonial awakening was conducted on the Gold Coast, Australia where the veil of the Divine Mother was removed to reveal her face. The energy of the Unnamed One emerged from a long silence to assist in the unveiling of the Mother. Now the Mother energy of wisdom and beauty, style and grace is available to envelop womanhood on planet Earth. The reunification restored the divine family connection into once more becoming a cohesive working team of divine order.

With the integration of these energies people are able to make the necessary shifts towards building more equitable communities. The divine energy is pouring through portals made available through Angel intervention. Scientists have labelled these openings as tears in the ozone layer. The tears will dissolve into tears as the Love energy dismantles the superior egos of those who consider they are the last word in explaining and controlling human endeavour.

Divine Father

As a lead player of divine energy on behalf of the family the Father was involved in many situations that had a direct bearing on human destiny. The will and drive offered as a benefit to human endeavour was converted into power. Now that the maleness he once fostered is no longer necessary he has merged back with the Mother energy. For the necessary shifting of the planet to take place the family of four becomes unified once more. It is the gift of the Rose symbolizing the Mother Energy that demonstrates the birthing of future events for the planet. The glorious story detailing the growth of Divine Womanhood will become a regular feature demonstrating an ongoing human future. In this coming and quickening of the dimensional upgrading the Father entwines and strengthens the Divine Mother energy.

Jésu

'What has been foretold will come to fruition. The memories from the past will come flooding to the surface.'

The energy known in entity form as Jésu first appeared on the planet some two and a half million years ago and has returned many times since then. Two thousand years ago he manifested onto this planet in a human form that is popularly recalled as Jesus, the bearer and fore-teller of Christos energy. It was not the first nor willed to be the last visit of one who relates to the title of 'The man of a thousand faces'. His planetary missions identified with the responsible guardianship of planet Earth and its adopted creatures.

When Jesus walked the planet two thousand years ago he spoke of the Divine Father in the cosmic sense and represented him as a player in cosmic Truth. It is small wonder that a religious people steeped in planetary cupidity, praying to a hillside god called Yahweh, should take exception to one who walked with so much cosmic energy and ridiculed their particular framed faith in god worship as just another form of paganism.

The Christos energy that represented through Jesus two thousand years ago is beyond planetary and even cosmic understanding. Such energy is nominated as eternal. Within it can be seen as androgynous or sexless. In expression, it is capable of taking on any form or persona. The character of Jésu as he is now known is a role-play destined to assist in transforming human consciousness from duality into oneness, from wilfulness into harmony, from separation into wholeness.

****

Lucifer

The other twin is known cosmically as 'The Unnamed One' though he carries many titles, one of which is the lordship of planet Venus. He is also instrumental in the further development of humankind, particularly to awaken areas of unconscious intelligence, dormant at present in the brain system of most civilized beings in societies.

The beyond cosmic entity/energy titled as Lucifer is an enigma for the minds of those who are ego driven as they are moved to contemplation. That the name is contained within the memories of human psyche is unquestionable. Yet the entity has never been on the planet in that name form though the energy has played many roles in the course of human history. At the time recorded in the Garden of Eden he was known as Adam. In Sumerian times he was called El. In the time of Jesus he played Simon Peter. Not least of all he played Sir Francis Bacon, scientist and co author with John Fletcher of the poems and prose writings of plays credited to William Shakespeare.

If the name of Lucifer is not portrayed in planetary memory then what has been recorded has been drawn from cosmic files. What is not obvious though to human minds that which is recorded has been drawn down by whom? Why do certain Christian church systems and Muslim religions rail against Lucifer, calling him an enemy and are fearful of his movements?

They were made aware of his close association with Satan or Sataan and erroneously linked the two energies as one though it is true the two are linked and working closely together with a like purpose. The Catholic fathers threw in the Devil for good measure, a creature of their own making as an extra to oppose their trinity of Jehovah, along with an iconic lacklustre version of Jesus and the Holy Ghost.

The Lucifer energy carries the torch of intelligence, bringing into light a greater understanding of illumination that eliminates the lesser lamps or candles of spiritual ignorance, which is rife amongst those observing religious faith. The Unnamed One signifies Lucifer as the titled bearer of the Torch of Intelligence. It is the light that shineth brightly as we work with Love and Intelligence to clear away the falsity imbedded in misshaped understandings in social education called knowledge and welcome in a New Mind, a New Day, into a New Dimension.

Chapter V.

The Cosmic Twins

The Jésu energy/entity enters through Jézel in 2004 to speak of wretched beings and to share in our discussion. Lucifer is telepathically advised of the theme in that instant and asks the lead in question.

Lucifer: Hello, brother. Have you got a hand for your brother?

Jésu then addresses the small gathering

Oh, Wretched Being

Oh wretched being
How was it that I did not recognize you
On that summer evening many moons ago
How was it that I passed you by
How can it be so
When I walk through the shadows
What now can I do?

Somewhere in myself I do recognize
Somewhere deep inside me
Something so strong

That I cannot put my hand out
To offer you a good day
And in so doing give myself the good day

Oh how I would yearn and yearn
For that summer evening many moons ago
When romance was in the air
Romance not of the popular variety
That is pronounced today
Romance in the connection
Romancing the connection
We did not need to touch
But I felt you so

And now I walked by you that other day
As though I did not see you
Because there is pain in it
For when I recognize you
I would then recognize myself
Oh wretched being, that will continue
Long after everyone puts the lights out

Hoodwinked, I hear you say
No, deep inside is that pulse
The yearning, the vibration
Of the ripples in the water
It is ready, it is there
When you put your hands out
And recognize ME

Each of you has been brought here
By the guiding hand of the Mother
It is she who bade me to say

*This verse for you this evening
Indeed I come not for myself
I come to do her offering
As you, each of you, are to do*

Lucifer: And will do

Jésu: That is to me the same thing

Lucifer then takes the centre stage to endorse his brother, Jésu, in offering their combined message.

*It is necessary for people
In this group to understand
Areas of work that are beyond them
Unless they take the hand*

*I like people who say of Lucifer
That fine wine addles his brain
So they may appear in superior strain
As to how he reads each picture
While from the red wine they abstain
They are caught in webs of stricture*

*I stand as a poet and with my pen
Compelled to utter and write again
Testing and tasting of your wen
Which of the Mother's children
Are to become Sataan acolytes then
Thus we in calling a rune a spade
Stand subject to agreements made*

*Lucifer stands as a poet of rote
I test you, I taste the essential you
That is why I am bound to quote
What is to be brought into view*

You who are of the Mothers' delight
Yes, you who are a Sataan acolyte
Sworn subjects to agreement given
Give over so you may be shriven

Discussion

Lucifer: There is one thing to say about dying: it means that you move into another level of energy. Where there is the dying…in the case of when the Angel energy takes over the body situation…there is a difference in that form of dying. Where an Angel takes over the body formation, there is the release of soul and you as a planetary self are out.

Who gave the vehicle of human life, the body system, which includes the ego dictated mind, the right to say it is they who are the dominant feature of the system? When did that happen? Yet you all buy the same story. You queue up at the same bloody bookstore to have the autographed book on your life assigned across to you. When will you acknowledge that you are not the body? You who are not of the mind never can be the body, and that is your ache within. There is your pain, because you attempt, you struggle, to be something that you cannot be. Oh, wretched being.

Lumley: What do you mean by wretched?

Zee: Fucked to the eyeballs.

Lucifer: *Laughing.* Wretched being simply means you are living in a continual state of unhappiness. You are immersed in a state of illusion, which does not allow you to locate the balance you are entitled to enjoy within yourself. Who in the room is prepared to take the hand of Jésu?

Birthing of Lucifer

Never has there been a poetic mind of such magnitude and understanding of human maladjustment since the days of Shakespearean plays and verse. The Angels call him Lucifer, a given title, which indicates the light of the torchbearer, the one who carries the understandings of cosmic intelligence to be shared amongst the multitudes grasping for a deliverance of future arrangements.

Lucifer is bonded within the Great Mother energy. The One has gifted him with the Grael of Intelligence maintained in **Truth**, **Equality** and **Unity**. The Great Dragon has invested a tongue to spread the flames of fire. The Shining Ones, Los Diabolos, the Lords of Lightning, bequeath to him a sharing of their combined strength. They will have him bring through new levels of light and life amongst the planetary creatures initially known as Man.

Through a series of internal and out of body experiences the Angels put Lucifer through absorbing courses of self-realization. Entity/energy visitations, which were experienced in the first three years, have enhanced the early psychic abilities to levels of atonement that can be described as reaching for a star setting beyond cosmic dimensions.

Here is a mini recall of exchanging entities 28 years ago.

One morning, it was a Wednesday morning as I remember in the early part of 1994, at approximately 11 o'clock in the morning, a man in his late fifties called Bruce sat alone at a downstairs table. He was attempting to write creatively on other world matters that for the last few months had been psychically intruding into his everyday awareness.

Meanwhile his wife had gone shopping in the nearby town of Caboolture. Suddenly, in his inner mind's eye, he saw a vision of her being killed in a traffic accident. Without a moment of thought, his reaction was simple. 'Do not take her', he exclaimed instantly, 'take me'. In that same instant whoever it is that overviews and organizes such areas of life and death exchanges on the planet accepted the offer.

Simultaneously, in the town of Caboolture, southeast Queensland, Australia, a loaded gravel truck swerved in the main street just in time to avert a potentially fatal collision, thus allowing his wife to live. Back at their house the man went immediately into a highly charged emotional death sequence that lasted some forty minutes while the soul occupying his planetary body exited from its hollow encasement and left this planetary system to journey Homewards.

Yet his mind and body still remained intact as a living breathing structure. The mental sensations of leaving, a regret of not saying goodbye to his family, a flood of tears and groans, which were caused in the process of the soul leaving, were too strong to deny the departure of the inner essence. Yet some part of his remaining mental energy was asking as to why the mind and body should not follow through a certain death situation by collapsing immediately?

Awakening to a New Mind

When he came once more into some conscious sense of recovery he was amazed to find that in the traumatic upheaval of the dying period where tears streamed so copiously that he had no ability to see, subconsciously he had written down on paper some beautiful lines in verse or song proclaiming his returning Home.

Going Home

So far away
Across the seas
My heart still lies
I know no ease
So I must go
Farewell, my friend
Yet I know we will meet
At our journey's end

So please don't cry
Don't mourn our loss
I cross a stream
We all must cross
Tell them I've reached
The mountain bold
My spirit's strong
The cross is pure as gold

I'm going home
Don't sigh for me
I've walked the land
I'll cross the sea
To all my friends
I leave behind
I promise I will wait
Seek, ye too shall find

This poem/song identifies an early part of a much bigger story waiting to be unfolded on the planet. It is a recounting of an energy exchange where two personas came to be sharing the same body for a short period of time. One soul having completed its contracted sojourn on this planet was required to lift out, while another entity, far greater in its span of energy level, dropped from the star system of Sirius into the vacated human system. As it is recorded in the memory banks of psyche I am able to relate the sensations of that distinctive period.

In the following weeks extending into months and then years there were indeterminate and confused areas of melding together a new form of living arrangement with a different set of understandings while breaking apart and dismissing a number of mental ego frames that certainly required replacing, as a prelude to an upgrading of cosmic intelligence.

The mental regrets of losing a worldly family were soon allayed for that initial confusion of self was sorted out to be followed by a realization of an expansive involvement in a magnificence of cosmic adventure in living matters of light that are still to come into fullness of being.

With the arrival of the new entity/energy there came a flood of intense feeling, a sensation of joy through experiencing an awareness of being part in a specific cosmic awakening that will shatter old worn out patterns of planetary conformity. There was a realisation of acquiring the assistance of Angels and many other cosmic entity/energies in delivering a greater uplifting in conscious awareness for people on Earth.

The progression of advanced cosmic work to be performed amongst people was not easily or readily forthcoming, more like a drip feeding of implanted understanding where information began to be relayed in various methods that induced forms of mental expansion. At times it felt like the head was being swollen, pressing against an imaginary steel band encircling the forehead.

The unnamed entity that now is seated firmly in the human system recalls the incidents where here were hard yards to do in assimilating the fresh energy into the body to acclimatise with the surrounding atmospheric pressure. Within the physical form there were also inherited planetary memory banks along with any amount of tenuous mind frames of ego distortion that badly needed some necessary readjustment.

Christos Light

***Jesus** said, 'What I do you shall also do and more.'*
'To find the Life let the outer become as the inner'.

Jésu as the bearer of the Christos energy carries in his heart the awakening of true life for all people. Each person carries the potential Christos energy within their being. It is the light that issued from darkness yet carries no shadow.

The Christos strain is the greatest form of energy the people on planet Earth will have the opportunity to experience in human form. For the next 10 to 15 years Jésu will make available greater levels of shared understanding to those who have ears to listen and eyes to see. These are not religious beliefs coming from us. Plus we have no interest in doubts.

The return of Jésu to this planet can be a reasonably scary experience for those who have always worshipped Jésu as an icon. This energy, which demonstrates the clarity of Christos energy, is not an icon. The energy goes far beyond planetary and even cosmic levels. To feel the energy that is in rapport with you and moves your very essence to awaken to Love is a beautiful experience we have no hesitation in calling realization.

The energy known in entity form as Jésu first appeared on planet Earth some two and a half million years ago. It was part of a team known cosmically as the 37 and was instrumental in getting the species of man who were crawling on their bellies to stand on two feet.

Different players of that initial team have returned many times. In Sumerian times, many thousands of years ago, the Jesus energy was known as Baal. Two thousand years ago he walked the planet as Jesus, the forecast bearer of the Christos energy. Now the energy is returning once more to support the timely rearrangement of life on planet Earth and once more to embrace the people of planet Earth in a greater understanding of Love energy.

Endowed once more with the name of Jésu to complete the full cycle of events, the energy will use the human system of a female called Jézel. Her designated work is to telepathically convey cosmic messages of benefit regarding the future purpose this world carries in a lead role for a cosmic shift of grand proportions. Initially, these messages of importance in human growth will be understandable to those who have their eyes already open and the ears to listen. Regardless of the denials from those who are materially and spiritually cemented into everyday belief patterns the people throughout the world will become intrigued and cannot help but be affected as they become more and more absorbed within the energy of **LOVE**.

It is the message Jézel carries that is important to be heard, absorbed and understood as she represents Divine Energy. She carries a deliberate energy that is of a divine strain. It is a divinity moving by design to shift the levels of present day human consciousness into a new dimensional area of greater significance. The strain she carries is a royal blue though some may see it as red.

It does not require the burdened load that accompanies the falsity of gods demanding worship from their followers. Religions with their rigmaroles of pomp, traditional ceremonies and rituals are collapsing and thus departing from the human arena as they are shifted elsewhere in the cosmos.

In their stead there will arise a new level of communal beings dedicated to three principles of **Truth, Equality,** and **Unity**. These principles and understandings are part of the new children being born on the planet today. To quote some previous words spoken by Jésu, 'A little child will lead them'.

Jésu is bringing through the Christos energy to engender a life-giving foundation for an energy that is not mentally disposed; rather the flow in its fullness will break open or apart the closeted human heart.

Christ consciousness is a development arising from divine energy that massages into memory the internal heart of all being. In sequential patterning Christ consciousness will overlap cosmic consciousness and simultaneously there is to be an exchanging of batons.

That which we offer in cosmic consciousness is required to include a section on embracing Christ consciousness. The Christos energy is formless and therefore cannot be framed into religious words that have the making of moral sense. Jézel has seen the energy many times as a smooth liquid with no lines. Lucifer has experienced the shivering sensation that aligns with the opening of the heart. He calls it a free flow of Love energy that is opportunely stored in the brain for future release. It was revealed to him as a secretion, green in colour, which will emanate throughout the nervous energy streams coursing within the human system.

Lucifer Experience

Jézel: There is beauty in the Christos energy. So I would like you to speak on what you encountered when you had the thrill of that energy in your system. Would you consider it was beauty that came up from the depth of your being?

Lucifer: In the experience there was beauty and with that feeling I shook uncontrollably. If the shaking had not occurred I might have been complacent about what was happening as I made an isolated phone call to an unknown woman who I decided to ring on what I considered was a whim. But because I did shake like a person being suddenly encased in ice on a hot summer's day in December...it occurred on the date of my birthday...what else could I do, but attribute the beautiful feeling of joy permeating my being to Love?

Jésu, the bringer or bearer of the essence we call Christos Energy, will open the hearts of people to the realization of Love. It is not that Lucifer does not carry Love, or understand Love, that he is not capable of delivering Love, but his area of work is Intelligence. The area of work for Jésu is the involvement of people in Love, pure and simple.

Jésu: I am here on the planet to promote and demonstrate a level of energy nominated as Christos, that which surpasses anything that cosmic understanding can comprehend. I will bind in the areas of Love energy through the promotion of the Christos energy on behalf of the Great Mother Energy.

Let those who have declared themselves as Christian throughout the last two thousand years now accept that the one they honoured is amongst them once again on planet Earth. Let them defer in honour of the one who brought Love into being onto the planet. And not only the Love he brought with him two thousand years ago this time he brings a greater level of energy, which we nominate as the Christos light, an emerging Love that is beyond any imagination of the total cosmic scenarios.

The Divine Mother endorses the Christos energy. She does not formulate its energy. In other words the energy does not come solely from the Great Mother. The Great Mother is involved because of the energy, any energy out of the Great Ocean. She is not divorced; she is part of. At this stage of cosmic development the Christos energy is separate only for the purpose of its own evolvement.

The light that Lucifer has brought forth and offers to those who are ready to embrace and forward our enterprise is only half a light. Now his brother, Jésu and his raiment of Christos energy moves in harmony with the light and the principles of **Truth Equality**, and **Unity** will break through. The Christos energy will walk arm in arm with greater understanding.

Love will rejoin and entwine to return our efforts to purposely serve the wishes of the Great Mother. It is the marriage of true minds or the two halves of the one heart that are being joined. In the marriage and the joining, they resolve that there can only be One. So with that understanding we return our pledge back to those who initially sent us forth.

Discussion with Jésu and Lucifer

20th November 2004

Jésu and Lucifer on behalf of the Divine Mother begin an initial group setting for Divine Womanhood entitled 'Getting to know you'. The following is an excerpt from their first gathering.

Lucifer: I have to say, because we are sitting in hallowed company this evening, that each of you carries a level of energy that very few people in polite society can aspire to. I would go so far as to say you are not human except in the planetary molded form of mind and body. Each of you instinctively knows that you come from a level of cosmic energy that is greater than what you experience in this daily grind in society.

So you wear masks and you maintain a pretence that you are the same or similar, just like everyone else. Yet we are aware that you are not. So it is my pleasure to introduce to you tonight the host of our gathering, Jésu, whose painted image appears over the fireplace. For those who have not checked it out already, we are welcoming back or in after two thousand years the level of energy that became known as Jesus Christ.

The promise Jesus made that he would return is now being made in the actual or the factional sense. We do not want to occupy you with thoughts of where we come from or what we know, except to say that we are not religiously bent or distorted. The energy of Jésu is not religious.

Jesus is not responsible for the spread of Christian faith. What we aim to do on planet Earth with the support of people of those of like mind will not revolutionize the planet or its people. We are aware human consciousness is to be moved to a new level of understanding known as the Fifth Dimension. We are skipping past the fourth, because it is a mud hole; it is swamp country and it is no longer necessary for human edification.

So tonight you are going to have the opportunity to talk with Jésu. We invite you to ask as many questions as you wish, and we do not care if you are sceptical. You may wish to be. It holds no interest for us because we are not interested in proving anything. We are interested in creating a new mind, a new day, and a new dimensional life for human benefit. Having said that, I am happy for Jesus to say that which is of further importance for greater understanding.

Jésu: Hello and welcome everybody, and thank you for coming to a Montecristos gathering. Yes, we are heralding in a new era. It is a new era of intelligence, a new era of enduring relationship. It is a new era, of each becoming cosmic and interacting accordingly with the people around you. To be able to go into future situations without the fear and trepidation that besets each of you now. Do not tell me that you do not have some trepidation in meeting different people and associating with them in an intimate fashion. It is possible to do that and not just with your so-called partner. How about with everyone? That is what we are heralding in, a new era of enduring relationship. A new era of understanding yourself, learning about, discovering who you are, and your interaction with various people. You do not fool me with your surface talk, the polite pleasantries. Many of you can do that blindfolded.

'Hello, how are you this evening? Isn't it nice we have had some rain this evening? And what do you do for a living?' Now we have moved past the trivia what do we say now? Is it more pleasantries or do we get into the areas of talking about your **self**, and who you really are? How often do you get into discussing that? How many of you do that? What would you like to see occur in the next 15 years. Not just with yourself, but with the people around you, those that are important in your life.

Then there are people in other continents, like the people in Iraq, the people in America, the people on the Ivory Coast in Africa, or is it that you don't care what occurs in these countries? I am not asking you to care about what the people are doing in these countries. I am asking you to be aware and to consider because in consideration, and looking into the different scenarios, you will find hidden areas within yourself.

It is called exploration. So this is what we nominate as 'Getting to Know You'. It is about an exploration of being. Exploring extremities, exploring areas most people would do well not to closely look at. Yes, they would be happy to have a dating agency or meet people occasionally in the pub. Casual talk, surface talk. Are you ready for the areas of exploration, the rivulets, the rivulets coming from the stream?

Lucifer: I thought rivulets went into the stream.

Jésu: They go into the stream, and they also come from the stream.

Lucifer: I am just attempting to get other people warm enough to respond and hit you with questions you cannot answer.

Aria: My question is why is it when you go out to mix and mingle with people that you have to smoke, do drugs or get drunk to be able to walk up and talk to people?

Jésu: Well, you are still carrying the mud of society, are you not?

Lucifer: I thought you were accusing Jésu of that, or are you talking about yourself?

Aria: I am talking about myself. I know when I go out and I see people they are on ecstasy, they are stoned, or they are drunk and I see that there is a game play going on. So to walk in and exchange with such people is really difficult. That is an area I have walked, and I am still walking.

Jésu: I say to you do not go where you are not welcome. There are areas on this planet where you are not welcome. Why tread those areas? Why, when you are still carrying the mud of those areas. You are already contaminated.

Eric: You travel those paths because you are looking for companionship, a sharing. That is why you go into those areas.

Jésu: I tell you she has not travelled the areas inside herself. She has not looked at the rivulets I am speaking of.

Eric: That is not an answer.

Jésu: Who said I was going to answer to your liking?

Eric: What is the purpose of the question?

Jésu: Maybe you have to ask yourself that. What are you looking for?

Eric: The answer.

Jésu: To?

Eric: To the question. *Lucifer starts laughing.*

Jo: What was the question? *She is laughing also.*

Eric: The question was why you have to travel these paths and do drugs and smoke, to gain association or relationship or whatever it might be.

Voice: Why should we have to keep away from those areas? Is it because we don't smoke or drink or whatever? Why should we have to be alienated from anywhere?

Another voice: You do not have to keep away. The question was why you have to do that to be able to talk to people. You can be there without doing it and talk to people.

Susannah: Let the energy talk. I mean answer please because she asked the energy.

Lucifer: It is not just any energy, it is Jésu.

Susannah: Then Jésu, please answer.

Lucifer: Well, it is an entity/energy. What I am saying is that it does acknowledge a name.

Jésu: Thank you. I had not finished speaking with...can you state your name please?

Eric: Eric is my name.

Jésu: Eric, thank you. It is important not to seek that which is considered yours outside of yourself, because self discovery comes from within. You can go into experiences, but it is not necessary. You are then being forced into further pain and dilemma.

Lucifer: What is being said there: if you are going to use the habits of other people to reflect what you would like to be or have done you are doomed to disappointment. Your peace and your understandings in life come from within you. It does not come from the reflection of other people's habits. What we say is the reflection for consideration is provided outside of you.

Jésu: Yes, that is correct. I say you are not to search outside of yourself for that which is inside you. Yes, of course, spend time with people, but to go into clubs and pubs, to go looking for ready made loose companionship is to find more pain, not companionship.

Zee: However, only through pain can you find yourself, so again there is a paradox. Yes, to a large degree people have to go outside; they have to be out there and have the experiences for themselves.

Jésu: I tell you the people here have gone through the experiences they are required to go through. None of you is required to go through any more so-called new experiences. I say this to each of you. Yes, you are to meet with different people. Yes, you are to see the reflection, but what has been asked, is not what you are saying.

Lucifer: The question each of you should ask yourself: when is enough pain sufficient? Why would you want to go out there and take on more pain?

Zee: The very fact that we carry ego, that is pain, and to release the ego you are to release the pain. To release something you have to go into it and through it.

Robin: Where does the pain come from? Who said pain?

Zee: Who said pain? *Laughing.* The very fact that you are in this dimensional atmosphere you are into pain regularly. Okay, I have to talk about myself. Yes, I am in pain because I am in this dimension. I have known this since I was little.

Lucifer: The atmosphere creates a pressure band that causes pain in the human system. Anyone who does not understand that the atmosphere puts pressure on the human system really has not looked at what circumstances surround them daily. What puts the emotional pressure onto the backs of people is society. Do you want to be a young girl and open the flick pages and see all those airbrushed models that tell you they are so much more beautiful than you? It is in every female type magazine, is it not?

Susannah: Yes.

Lucifer: And if you meet those people in so-called real life and you think, hang on, can this freckled face person who lacks uplifted boobs be this absolutely glamorous thing that appears on the pages of a magazine.

Voice: There is nothing wrong with freckles.

Lucifer: *Laughing.* Okay, I stand corrected. What I am saying is that the glamour displayed in society flicks is a sham. When you attempt to catch hold of glamour it disappears as if it were fairy floss. Who can get lasting satisfaction out of admiring or eating fairy floss? Can fairy floss replace a meal that will sustain you? No, it cannot, and glamour portrayed in society will not sustain you either.

****

Jésu: I would like to mention the requirement to break the shell. People consider that breaking the shell makes one vulnerable and open to the miseries and the powers of other people. It is a misconception. When you are breaking the shell of ego, yes, there is a phase of being neutral

The Cosmic Twins

like between changing gears, then moving into the next gear, which is called cosmic. Therein lies the strength. The strength is always inside you, but you cannot see it because you are focused on the glamour out there.

What is out there? That is why I say to you, you will never find what you seek out there. You will see the reflection, but you will not find yourself out there. You may search day in and day out and you will not find yourself out there. So to break the shell, first see yourself like the little chicken in the shell.

When are you ready to come out into the open? When are you ready to expose yourself for who you really are? Each of you here is wearing a mask. You put on the appropriate mask for the moment to say this is what I am going to present to each person. An unmasking is required, a breaking of the shell, and that is what we are to do.

Eric: Does everybody in this room wear a mask?

Jésu: Yes, indeed.

Eric: Including you?

Jésu: Yes.

Lucifer: Jésu in itself is an entity, it is not the energy.

Jésu: Jésu is a name. A name has been given to the person of two thousand years ago, what you in English-speak call Jesus. I am not Jesus as such.

Lucifer: I was saying last night that Jésu or the energy behind Jésu is also mentioned in the Bible amongst the Canaanites. In Sumerian times he was known as Baal. *Jésu breaks into laughter* He is an old associate of Jehovah.

Jésu: Very well known. So Eric, you have some things to say.

Eric: I always have a lot to say.

Lucifer: That is why you have that choke in your throat.

Eric: How do I remove it?

Jésu: By writing the letter. Poetry may well be your forte.

Eric: Maybe the talent that is in there is still yet to develop.

Lucifer: And it is also our promise. For those of you who wish to step into your next level of understanding of who you are, we will show you undisclosed areas of yourself that you can experiment with. When you reach the point in your life where you say, 'I no longer wish to be part of the old ways' then we will show you an area within you that will allow you to strike out as a pioneer, to create something afresh or new that the unawakened people in society have not yet experienced.

Jésu: Each of you has a gift, unopened as yet. You still have the ribbons tied. So Eric, are you ready to look at the gift?

Eric: When you reach the stage that I am at in my life where I have come through the troubles, the torment, and the anguish. You want me to go back through all those troubled times and relive the pain?

Jésu: No, that is not necessary. It is very important for everyone to understand that there is camaraderie and joy available beyond the third dimension on this planet. Realize that you have been dipped into the swamp, the planetary area referred to as painful, which comes from the pressure of this third dimensional plane. There is available, camaraderie beyond what people are calling friendship here and there is joy within to share.

Lucifer: And there is Love within that supports all things.

Susannah: Two thousand years ago Jesus went around, and spoke thus to people.

Jésu: He certainly did. *Laughing.*

Susannah: They felt something. They had a connection. They felt the love. They felt something.

Jésu: Did they?

Susannah: Why not? We feel it now. Why not you give us something to lean on, something we can hold on to. We cannot run. We have to stand up and start to walk, to put one foot in front of the other and start to walk. When we can walk, when we are stable, then we can run. From what I understand now, you are asking us to run foremost.

Lucifer: No, I did not hear that. We do not ask you to run. We ask you to first sit still.

Susannah: Yeah, I do that. Yet I do not feel anything here. I don't feel any love of what we are supposed to feel here.

Lucifer: You are lucky if you are not feeling anything. Then you are ahead of the group.

Susannah: I wasn't there two thousand years ago.

Lucifer: You weren't? How do you know that?

Susannah: I can't remember that.

Lucifer: That does not mean you were not there.

Susannah: Okay, I can't remember that. I have knowledge from films and books that Jesus was sparkling with love and you felt something. Why is it you can't give us something, something to live with now?

Jésu: Let me tell you that two thousand years ago for the majority of the time it was hard yakka.

Susannah: What happened two thousand years ago?

Jésu: You closed yourself down and you are still closed down.

Susannah: Nothing has changed.

Jésu: *Yelling.* You are still closed down.

Susannah: Yeah, I do that. You should not yell.

Jésu: Who told you that?

Susannah: Why do you have to take your voice up?

Jésu: So you can hear what I am saying to you. You are talking without listening. Your ears are closed.

Susannah: Tell me something so I can open them up.

Jésu: Giving needs to be without wanting advantage. Love exudes without intent. It is inside everyone. For you to feel, the flame of Love is to be opened up inside of you. At this moment you are overloaded with doubts and fears.

Susannah: It is inside every one of us. I do not feel anything.

Jésu: Yes, because you carry emotional baggage. It is the attachment to those around you. You are a needy person. You need something from somebody else. Until you learn to find strength inside you, you will continue to have this hole.

Susannah: I know that and understand that, which I try to do. Still I have no **thing** to hang onto to go further.

Jésu: Great. I do not wish you to hang on.

Lucifer: Take your fingers off what you have already held fast and you will move through.

Jésu: You are carrying a full cup, and that is why you cannot hear what is being said. You come here with a full cup. You are to empty it.

Susannah: How?

Jésu: You speak of what is in the cup and let it go. Realize it is no longer of use.

Susannah: I am hanging on to everything. I need what I have for some reason, even the pain. It is my pain. I deserve this pain.

Lucifer: Actually it is not yours.

Susannah: I think it is mine.

Lucifer: It is not. It is the DNA drip feed coming from your ancestors.

Susannah: Okay, but how would I know that?

Lucifer: You will find it out.

Susannah: When? *The history blocking her past memory is that she played Caiaphas, the head priest of the Sanhedrin responsible for the Jewish agitation that put Jesus on the cross.*

Jésu: Allow what is being said to you and do not file it anywhere. Your ego mind will say, 'this is of advantage, this I can use and this I can't use'. Instead allow what is being said to you, rather than wanting instant answers. That which is important is inside you, so you will not find satisfaction from what I say to you. All that is required is for you to allow the energy within you to stir, to have willingness.

Susannah: Convince us with something. Tell us something, tell me something, or show us the way. How can we give it up, and start again from zero with nothing from nowhere, and go to the unknown without anything to support us.

Lucifer: Okay, are you ready to listen to me? Acknowledge your beauty.

Susannah: Nothing. It has no meaning. I am waiting for some answers, a miracle.

Lucifer: Of course there is no meaning. The tears are very close. Acknowledge your beauty within and you will have the breakthrough and there is your miracle.

Susannah: I do not need my beauty. What do I need that for? What is that for? What is beauty?

Robin: What do you need a miracle for?

Susannah: To break the shell. The shell that she/he told us to break.

Lucifer: Actually, Jesus in his present role is male.

Susannah: Yes, okay.

Lucifer: Acknowledge your beauty and you will have your miracle. Can you not see that?

Susannah: I cannot. I have been seeking many, many things for many years. Shit keeps coming up, back to me all the time. When am I going to realize I am so beautiful?

Lucifer: You are looking for a physical situation. We do not speak of these matters in the physical sense.

Susannah: Okay, I understand that, but still there is nothing.

Jésu: I would like to ask you a question. Would you like to meet with the Mother?

Susannah: I didn't understand the question. Whose mother?

Jésu: The Mother of all us here, the Divine Mother.

Susannah: Yes, why not? Yes.

Lucifer: Do you want time out to write a list of past complaints before you meet with her?

Susannah: Okay, yeah, show me the way. Tell me what to do. Do I follow her?

Jésu: When you wish to meet her then we can make some time with you.

Susannah: Okay, agreed.

Lucifer: So we start a journey with one step.

****

Eric: Where does trust and faith come into play?

Jésu: Trust and Faith? Okay, it is inaccurate to say that I did not yell two thousand years ago. I was not enamoured of many people. Many people ridiculed Jesus. They were involved in revenge, deceit, and advantage. And you are seeing a replay happening today. Are you prepared to sit here and allow without quibbling? Are you prepared to do the hard yards on yourself? I tell you that you will not get there through trust; you will not get there through faith, and you will not get there through worshipping Jesus.

Lucifer: And forget about hope. We will throw that one in. You can give hope a miss also.

Voice: How about belief in yourself then?

Jésu: No, also forget belief in yourself. Belief is a lie given to you by family, friends, and teachers. I do not believe in myself. What significance is there in that? How can that assist you? You say 'this is who I am', and it is not so. It is a role play, it is an act, and your whole life has been a series of acts. Let it all go.

Voice: Okay, you throw everything out. Then what?

Jésu: Then you will see that which is left is knowing. That which is innately you. Attempt to throw it out and it will remain. At this stage, you do not know who you are, and what is not you. It is all mixed in together.

To put trust in somebody requires that you do not trust somebody else. Therefore there is mistrust with any number of people. How can you work with people and have an understanding of people if there is mistrust? Do you not understand that if there is a trust placed in somebody then with somebody else there has to be mistrust? It has to even out on this planet. Good or bad is only perspective the same as trust.

****

We are going into a beautiful section of history for humankind. In present times it may appear to be devastating, horrific, and sad, with all of those areas of man killing man and cruelty to others. Nasty energies are afoot, but it is like an implosion of disruptive energy and disintegrating rapidly.

It appears to be man fighting man, but it is an implosion happening inside people. It can also be seen on a country level, and inside everyone there is a shift of energy occurring. The upheaval in and around you is like a roller coaster. People are not able to balance their selves. But I tell you they will not want to go that extra distance, and it is available to go that extra distance. More is still to come in the next 15 years.

Let go of every **thing**. You see the mind is already saying what it can hold on to because the mind is acquisitive. You will now be considering, 'okay, what can I hold on to then. It doesn't seem right that I can let go of everything, because I will have nothing. I am going to be nobody.'

Voice: For me once you let go of everything then where do you go from there?

Jésu: We go into the next gear, a new life mode. Why are we here? We are here to enter into this beautiful era I have been speaking of. We are here to assist humans to go through this rocky period, and to assist them we first have to go through the rocky period ourselves.

Lucifer: So each person sitting in this room is a pioneer of sorts, whether you kick, whether you scream. Just because some kick and scream occasionally, and they have to be removed as recalcitrant children does not mean they are not going to do the work. They will do the work.

I tell you some people have no liking for the words of Jésu, because in their minds Jesus two thousand years ago did not validate them. So this time in a perverse manner they are going to do their damnedest to show Jesus they will not step and validate him. What do you call it, tit for tat?

Jésu: Yes indeed. *He is laughing.* What is being offered is food for consideration.

A Tribute to the Indomitable Spirit, Lucifer

Indomitable Spirit

Indomitable Spirit, Lucifer, dressed as man
How wide is the measure of your wing span
Do tell us of your image; how it has grown
Since you ascended to the worldly throne
What has become of the natural mien to be
When first you crossed the deep blue sea
What of your plumage, do colours prevail
Now you have entered into this sorry tale
Give out with the stories, tell us your plan
Invite down our destinies as only you can
We wait in suspense, Shade, dressed as man

Chapter VI.

Greater Council of Nine

Discussion with the Greater Council of Nine

9th January 2015

In the Wednesday evening discussion, Lucifer had requested the Greater Council of Nine to give us confirmation of our future part in the Divine Plan. The greater energy takes the opportunity to make contact.

Unnamed: I would like to say to you very clearly, we are of the Unnamed. We come to you this evening to tell you of future happenings. We are compelled to say to you that the movement into the Fifth Dimension is happening as we speak. Most folks, maybe yourselves, will have noticed nothing different, but maybe there are one or two of you that have noticed a shift into the Fifth Dimension. If you have then you are well on your way to realising a New Day. A New Life.

Life on this planet, as you are aware of it, is numbered, as many folk know it is numbered. The Fifth Dimension is coming through onto this planet and as a consequence you will then see that a like energy is coming through on many other levels in the cosmic area.

The cosmic area is filled with a variety of dimensions; it is just not stuck on five or six or seven or whatever number you want to name. You who want to remain stuck in this dimension need to realise that we are moving. So let's be flexible. Let us be unnameable. Let's not name others with what you see is a weakness. If you are now considering others and their weaknesses you are in effect talking of your own.

So you who are still in this little grouping here require some adjustments. You still do not realise that what you see outside yourself is inside you. If you are okay with that all well and good, but if you are not then you need some adjustments. If you are not happy with those who sit here at this table then you need some further adjustment in your systems, because these are the ones that you are going to work with closely.

We who are Unnamed are giving you this update, this evening. Is it about honesty with what you see in others? Ah, it is a little bit more than that. It is a little bit more. It is unfinished business. Are you at fault because of this, would you say? Are you claiming religion or your upbringing because well religion and upbringing are synonymous? It doesn't matter whether you went to a religious centre, or if you did not, it was still religious input.

We are bringing this to you this evening because if you are to work together so closely, which will be required, you will need to be able to see clearly, not half-hearted prejudices because of your own upbringing. Yeah, everybody has certain misalignments and they are not a hundred percent in this or that area. Yes, correct, but does that stop you from working with them?

This is a very important and deep question that we ask of each of you. Are you prepared to look at it? And look at it seriously without saying, 'I am denigrating the other person and I won't look at myself because it is the other person at fault'. Nobody here in this group on this planet is perfect. Nobody! So forget the perfection.

You have, all of you, strengths that you are capable of using and that is what you are to look at and that is what you are to utilise. If, for example, you are to let go of those other petty areas then the strength will be even greater. We who are Unnamed will be of support to each of you that sit here this evening, but we will not support your silly biases towards each other in whatever fashion it so happens to call each of you on whatever moment or day.

That is not part of the Divine Plan. The Divine Plan says that each of you has to work towards cleansing your areas of weakness, which means that when you see each other and you claim that the other is weak or so inclined then you are to clean your own area. Not the one that you dislike in whatever format it arrives.

Awakening to a New Mind

We want that to go through your heads, thick or thin, as they may be. This is a very important message from those who are Unnamed. We don't want you to thank us. We don't want you to particularly acknowledge us. You come from us in proportionate measures. But if you consider that you are going to get away with nominating someone else in this arena as not fit, look at yourself. We will do the over viewing of those who sit here this evening.

There is another one coming through. Can you just be patient? Thank you.

Lucifer: We haven't had you in for a long time. Sataan, or the Great Dragon. The energy is synonymous.

Great Dragon: *The dragon makes hissing noises.* So events are unfolding quickly. Hello. Events are moving miraculously forward. No, I joke on miraculous; they have been many steps along the way. You who sit in this illustrious grouping; you are not special, but you have specialist work, each of you has specialist work ahead. Each of you will work in some way towards rewriting the history books.

But you have no ownership on your particular area. You might say that the Mother has given me this area of work, and that will be so, but that does not mean that others cannot have input into the area that you have been designated. That means each of you will cover all areas at different times.

You are not the be all and the end all of one particular area. But if others decide or realise that there is a message in there to extend or open an area then they are all welcome to put their input into that area. So you are all welcome. You, each of you, are all available to put your own areas into each of those areas. When I say your own input, we know that it is not planetary input; because if it was so it would not be useful.

Let me say that again: your reliance on planetary areas is not welcome. So that is a big factor in this work. If you are able to take that on board you will go the distance. Yes, I am saying that it is not still irrevocable that you are in here for the long haul. You may drop off at the last moment because you want to continue to put forth your planetary bias towards this or that person, whatever the case may be. *Pause.* Your next person is coming through.

The One: Hi guys. I have unduly been given a certain treat, a certain amount of kudos because I have produced an unending supply of what is called Intelligence. Now I know that I have been given that ability. So I don't take on the kudos, because if I were to take that on I would be a gone goose. So if you take on credit for your abilities to present whatever it is that you have been presented with, you are also in that area of gone goose.

The One speaks with you this evening. The One who has been given the keys to the door, if you like; The One that has been given the picture, the overall picture of life…not so much on this dimension, but life in a general phase. I have been given many views. But the most important of all is that I am steeped in the Love Energy, although I have not been given the ordinance to open that up.

I have been given the ordinance to open up Intelligence. I have been given the area of opening up your keys to your development, where each of you has an area that needs to be developed. You are not there yet. Some are closer than others.

Lucifer obviously has to be up top, and Jésu close behind. Not every one of you has to reach the zenith of intelligence. Not required, not necessary. And it does not mean that you are less than or better than in any way, shape or form, because that is not how the Great Mother and myself operate.

You may say what is in your minds, but that is only in your tiny third dimensional/fourth dimensional minds. We operate in conjunction with each other. We are in many ways one. We are unified; we sit in Truth. We are not separate as such. We have been moved into these distinct positions to acknowledge areas within the systems that will activate and then bring forth a merger. But that has not happened yet. So while that has not happened we will remain distinct from each other.

Lucifer: I have a question.

The One: Yes, sir, please proceed.

Lucifer: What I am hearing you saying is that Truth seats behind **Equality** and **Unity**?

The One: Yes sir, that is indeed so. Not that I said that, but you have picked that up. That is right on the dime. And that is not quite available yet, monsieur; it is not available yet. But those like yourself; you will start to bring onto this planet the diamonds that will deliver Truth to the doorsteps of each of those on the planet.

Lucifer: So my next question…if you are okay with me asking you these.

The One: We are more than happy to hear questions.

Lucifer: Okay; then what was presented to me yesterday was that the Unnamed have been keeping a seat warm for the Diamond Essence. And they are happy to step back or away and allow the Diamond Essence to take their position in the Greater Council of Nine. Is that accurate?

The One: What you are saying is futuristic. It has not happened yet. But to all intents and purposes, yes. This in your timeline here on this planet will be not far away, but no, it has not happened yet.

Lucifer: So it is portentous.

The One: That is correct. We have one more person to speak with you. Thank you.

Great Mother: And so good evening to each of you here.

Lucifer: Good evening, Mother.

Great Mother: You who are my children…you who have put yourself forth in my name. You who have represented yourselves as my **self**, you will then recognise and relate to the energy, which speaks with you now. You will feel the thread that passes between my **self** and each of you. So feel the thread of energy. That is enough to feel that thread of energy.

Let me say that I present for each of you. I do not denigrate you. I do not say you are lacking, because none of you are lacking; none of you are requiring of denigration. The denigration comes as it will from inside of you; that which is not related to the Great Mother. That part of you that still denies the Great Mother. So that which denies the Great Mother energy has to be brought forth into the light.

Lucifer: That has to be the will and the power of the dissident Father energy. And it has to be brought into view and it has to be exposed for what it is. That it is less than the generosity of Love, which is the foundation and support system of all cosmic life.

Great Mother: You see that area can easily be taken care of. Each of you is capable of doing that in your own manner. **Each of you is greater** than the male energy that purports to dominate certain aspects of this planet. Yes, it does do that. But you, my children, have been given the energy to go beyond that.

So I don't see that the father energy/male energy can stop any of you here. It can stop many, yes, but not any of you here. It can give you a little bit of angst or a little bit of pain. Yes, but not more than that. You have to move through those areas, and you have the energy to do that. The Great Dragon, The Unnamed, The One and myself have given you that ability, that opportunity to do that. And in so doing you can give that to others who are interested in moving through the father energy that has been given precedence on this planet.

Lucifer: So, Mother, please explain to us some form of understanding of the Diamond Energy.

Great Mother: The Diamond Energy is beautiful to behold, and within the Diamond Energy there is the Love Energy. But let me tell you I am not of that energy, although I am still in that energy. The Great Mother energy is beyond…

Lucifer: What I am asking simply is this: is the Diamond Energy the foundation of the Great Mother energy, or is it another form of intelligence that we are to absorb?

Great Mother: One of the intelligences that you are to absorb would be the correct response.

Lucifer: So the Great Mother is…

Dauphinia: Is beyond that.

Great Mother: I am in it, I am also beyond it. That is what I am saying to you.

Lucifer: I am hearing then, is Love still all embracing of each of these other great energies…?

Great Mother: Yes, until there is any further notice, that is it, forever and a day. *Laughter.*

Lucifer: I am okay with that.

Dauphinia: Finally.

Lucifer: Oh no, I mean these energies for Lucifer are meant to be understood. They present themselves tonight and they say we are here to help take you through.

Great Mother: Yes, I have some wine here. So I wish to say cheers to you, this could be…I am saying could be because it is up to you in some ways to make it bigger, but it is a turning point, and it can be bigger than that. You have to put yourselves forward to do that.

Lucifer: And we are prepared to do that.

Great Mother: Cheers. *Glasses clink.* I would like that you read what has been said very carefully. Not once, not twice, but a minimum of three times that you read through what each has said to you this evening. You are children of the Great Mother. Do not put that aside ever. That is foremost in your work here. The Fifth Dimension beckons. It is calling. Can you hear it?

Lucifer: Yes, I for one can.

Dauphinia: I can feel it; I can't hear it.

Great Mother: Same thing, feel, hear, whatever it takes, it is there presenting itself.

Lucifer: And as such we will present an ongoing presentation for those on the planet.

Great Mother: In that regard.

Lucifer: So that the people can get some understanding of what lies ahead of them in their future life.

Great Mother: Good evening to you all. Sweet kisses to you all.

Lucifer: And we are only too happy to receive your kisses.

Discussion with an Envoy of the Great Dragon

23rh June 2011

Notes as remembered prior to the tape being turned on.

Lucifer: What is happening with the **Big Boomers**?

Envoy: The Great Dragon is smoking the peace pipe with them.

Lucifer: What about the release of the finance?

Envoy: All in its time.

Lucifer: Is there something not happening inside of us that we can work with?

Envoy: Nature abounds.

Lucifer: The Little People are on the move.

They speak on the subject of Truth. Satania asks a question about Truth: 'is it not to be in confusion and then having found clarity Truth arrives'. The envoy does not respond directly. Instead he speaks about a shaft of light appearing.

There is discussion on the three principles and their preference for working with one area. Lucifer says Truth and Satania says Equality.

The tape is activated.

Lucifer: You are saying that there cannot be sound unless the quality comes forth in the rainbow light. Is that reflection being cast from the scales of the Great Dragon? Am I correct in saying that? Or do you prefer that in the movement of the Great Dragon the rainbow colours are projected or promoted?

Envoy: From the promoted, but we must include sound in that equation.

Lucifer: Well, the sound I hear from the Great Dragon is like the roaring of a bull.

Envoy: That which you hear is primal energy.

Lucifer: It is male.

Envoy: It is the initial scream that comes forth after the babe is born.

Lucifer: Is it not muted in the human child?

Envoy: A hundred fold.

Lucifer: Subdued.

Envoy: At least.

Lucifer: There is no celebration in the birthing, as there is no celebration in the death sequence.

Envoy: It is a cycle.

Lucifer: Life is like a practice plane that touches the ground momentarily before it lifts back off again. It is not meant to stay grounded. It was never meant to ground.

Envoy: You wear the joker's cap as one who speaks and establishes Truth. *The envoy coughs and we offer red wine, which is accepted and a mouthful is taken.*

Lucifer: Tell us about this joker's cap?

Envoy: You describe it.

Lucifer: You describe it, Satania.

Satania: You asked the question.

Lucifer: Yes, and you are entitled to put forward your idea.

Satania: It is like a jester's cap. So it is back to you now.

Lucifer: I see the joker as slightly different from the jester. I see the joker posing the questions that draw sanity out of stupidity. The jester does the same type of work.

Envoy: The difference is the joker has a smear on the face.

Lucifer: That sounds like my ancient trainers. (Satyrs) A sneer or a smear?

Envoy: A smear.

Lucifer: That looks like a sneer.

Envoy: Yes, looks like, but is not.

Lucifer: So what does the joker offer?

Envoy: Release.

Lucifer: So then the jester offers relief. In other words the people laugh for a little while and then fall back into their age old patterns.

Envoy: Pain.

Lucifer: And the joker can take them beyond the pain. *The envoy laughs without displaying amusement.* Very few humans would be comfortable linking with the joker.

Envoy: Very few.

Lucifer: But enough?

Envoy: Is that a question?

Lucifer: Of course. Like grist to the mill.

Envoy: Enough. You don't need to meet everyone.

Lucifer: When you say to meet you mean in effect well met. Not many, very few, are what we can call well met.

Envoy: Where did you get your style from?

Lucifer: *Laughing.* How far would I have to go back to the asking of that question? Or to provide an answer to the question?

Envoy: Ha ha. The latest in style.

Lucifer: Do you mean the style we wear today?

Envoy: That you wear in your speech.

Lucifer: My trainers have been so many. When I go back I cannot separate the words of the Great Mother and the Great Dragon. Though I know they separated for the cause of which we work with today. But it cannot possibly be that they were different or that they were less than one. When the initial rose was born, then the Dragon was also born. Am I not correct? Or did the Dragon precede the rose?

Envoy: The Dragon came with the teardrop.

Lucifer: With the teardrops. So the Dragon was formed out of teardrops?

Envoy: It came with the teardrop.

Lucifer: You see that is what I would have to consider unknowable.

Envoy: Tell me if you can see a tear drop on the rose petals.

Lucifer: Of course. We call it a dewdrop. Though whether the Dragon came from the tear drop or...

Envoy: With the tear drop.

Lucifer: To me that is still unfathomable.

Envoy: Let it be for now. Let it sink into your very being.

Lucifer: Was the Mother then weeping?

Envoy: Yes. Yes, if you prefer, teardrops.

Lucifer: Weeping for her lost children.

Envoy: Yes.

Lucifer: And from those teardrops Dragon energy was born?

Envoy: Yes.

Lucifer: So in what I painted as the rose being circumvented by the Dragon means that the rose was a latter conception.

Satania: I thought you just said that the Dragon came with the teardrop.

Lucifer: But the Dragon was already there when the rose burst into the cosmos. So the rose is a latter conception that has come from the Great Mother. So is the Great Mother a symbolic expression of the ocean? Or does that go further back again? What I am saying is that the womb of all being is the ocean and that we see the symbolic Great Mother representing that area.

Envoy: That is appropriate.

Lucifer: Because for our Intelligence, if you like, or at least our understanding of Intelligence we require a symbol...so a symbol that does not carry superiority.

Envoy: What is superiority?

Lucifer: The inclination to be seen as bigger, better, brighter, than others. It is an attitude.

Envoy: So what it is will go awry without the grace of the Mother.

Lucifer: However, I still see the pain built into the separation. Till we can conjoin the various areas within ourselves then people will still suffer from pain and continue to wear the pressure of separation. Not a very pleasant costume.

Envoy: The pressure will arrive at twilight.

Lucifer: The dawning of the fifth dimension?

Envoy: Each time you have the stabs of pain please join again with the teardrop until the dawning of that new plane arrives.

Lucifer: I am happy to wear what is seen as physical pain. I know that each time I work it through my system that I am in some way advancing the cause of Love.

Envoy: What each of you does will accord with moving through your obligatory areas of pain?

Lucifer: But I never thought when I saw the painting that Zee did with the roses and their dewdrops that each one of them was a Dragon tooth. I will look now at the painting in a different light. *The envoy smiles.* Have we completed our discussion?

Envoy: The Dragon carries all the elements in one.

Lucifer: When you say elements I understand that you mean to include the three principles, the Love and Intelligence. Also is there an area then that we have not understood that is carried by the Dragon? Would you see peace as an element?

Envoy: And smoking the peace pipe I mentioned earlier. Perhaps you could say that.

Lucifer: The Dragon doesn't quite fit the planetary image of peace. I could say that breathing fire and smoke and a tail that can spin the vines of...

Envoy: Make a whirlpool. A great disturbance in the mind. We are finished.

Lucifer: Thank you very much. Were we able to bless I would do so. *Lucifer moves across and takes the hand of the Envoy.* Instead I will receive the blessing.

Satania: Thank you. *Satania also takes the hand of the Envoy.*

Discussion with the Great Dragon

21^{sd} July 2014

Lucifer: The dragon's role is to move ahead of crises, shifting and clearing obstacles until each sequence of events come into some willing conformity. The dragon has the footprint, the One makes a cast. He sets it in stone. The Dragon requires the intelligence from the One to endorse the preliminary work.

Let us look at the bigger picture. What The One throws in front of the Dragon for review is distraught material. The planet has been overviewed by the universal creatures who came from similar areas we assign to the working of Ancients. They in turn were overviewed by the Uncles in the Divine Estate, whose work in turn were instated by The One and the Dragon utilizing their efforts to ensure that each section of the Divine Plan was instigated. In these areas you will find the beginning of chapters but not the beginning of the book. The Divine Plan is coming from where we are working towards returning and on our way we are to deal with matters requiring adjustments to ensure balance. So it is our work on the planet to realize what is meant to be settled.

It has been a prolonged action or activity to understand the weaknesses besetting character building. We have to keep going back to the Divine Plan for guidance. It was set up to research weaknesses in the strengths.

Great Dragon: The Great Dragon has a few words to say on the mishmash of what is called reality. What you realise is less than profound. The ideas that were put into your heads a long time ago were meant to confound what is ahead of you. For you to meet in equal terms is meant to propound understanding. Why were the species of humans initially built? Were they to be toys of cosmic design? That is a question requiring a response.

Jézel: No. The answer is no. However, they have been used as cosmic toys.

Great Dragon: Agreed. And you have to say that agreed can be broken apart to say that it is a form of greed. Why are human systems continuously developed? Obviously there has to be a purpose. Can any human nominate their purpose?

Jézel: No.

Great Dragon: Once again, we are in agreement. The future though mapped out is beyond human comprehension. The way forward is beyond their ability to meet life as it is meant to be interpreted. So does life have the ability to interpret its own future? We would say not. Humans are seen as children. Does the child tell the parents how they require their future developed understanding to unfold?

Jézel: No.

Great Dragon: Well, maybe in today's society you could possibly say the children have more call regarding involvement in environment than the parents are competent to supply. But of course a child does not have the sophistication of understanding that will allow them to meet adversity and fulfil prophecy, and allow that each of these enterprises are required to equalize.

The Great Dragon draws its understanding from a greatness of awareness that derives its philosophy from areas of advanced acknowledgement, which in its formal performance feeds understanding into cosmic levels that are appreciative.

We have no interest in supplying and supporting cosmic areas that have no interest in receiving fulfilment. We have no interest in those who still think that their earlier progression entitles them to maintain a future fulfilment.

The Great Dragon Energy is all about intelligence. It is prepared in that central feature to have acknowledged the opportunity of producing intellectual information. On the other hand it is adamant that what is Intelligence is not open to planetary interpretation, because any planetary interpretation is falsehood.

It cannot accentuate the intelligence because it has been bought and sold on behalf of those who see human activity as no more than slavery. That is all the Dragon has to say at this time. Obviously there will be more to be stated futuristically. That is enough for this evening.

Be advised that there are many more Greater Energy effects who are prepared to visit their comprehensive understanding upon the small world grouping of Lucifer and his cohorts. These will arrive systematically, so the understandings can be shared throughout human collateral.

Discussion with the Great Dragon

9th May 2019

Dragon noises are heard occasionally throughout the transcription.

Great Dragon: We come this evening to pay homage to the Great Mother. Yes, this planet is in a woeful condition. However, we must see that the planet is going through the death throes. Dragons do not see it as death. But because you understand death throes we will throw that saying into the ring. All ancient and modern methods are out of sync and therefore not useful in this period of the planet. So people can't go back to rely on tradition. They cannot go forward on the so called new age method. Neither is useful or appropriate.

We, the Dragon energy, are strongly an advocate for the Great Mother energy and hence Love is to infiltrate, permeate. But first you are to receive the blast of energy in shifting dimensions. It will work in various ways because of where you are at this stage in your development. If you are into the planetary system, it won't be the easiest of transitions. Anyway, you receive the news and the rearrangement first. And actually there may be one or two others. And one day you will get to meet those one or two others.

The sons are designated to present the proceeding development of planet Earth and so they are required to clear the slate for the availability of the next level to be opened up and shared. Shared!

There are no more hidden elements. Everything of the energy nature...Love must be shared and following on from that there is an appreciation of greater understanding.

So if you are aware or opening up in anyway, then you are required to put your developments, or your understandings, or your energy shift, whatever way, shape or form that is, on the table. The Angels won't do it for you. Certainly, the Mother will wait for you to come to her. Love waits. Intelligence sits patiently while the present mindsets are still running around in frantic circles.

When you come to understand the beauty within your system, the façades that you consider are keeping you safe will no longer be an issue. The guards you take on are old hat. They will no longer protect you. And the new mind that Lucifer is exposing will start to make its way into the system.

The kiss of the Dragon is with thee and Lucifer. I am one with the Great Mother.

Each takes the hand and the Dragon makes hissing sounds and groans as he sends kisses to everyone in the room.

Remembering

To be an anchor of the light
A star of wisdom in the night
A fount of water in the day
To those who thirst along the way
To see all things with clarity
Reminds myself of who we be
To set the measure of a mile
And lose it all in your smile
Accepting joy is all we need
Strengthens love, replaces greed
Then when our day of work is done
We are in peace, eternally one.

Chapter VII.

Cosmic Energy

Discussion with the Greater Energy

Bringers of Life
16th November 2012

Every **thing** visible in the cosmic sky is but a pale shadow reflecting from those of the Greater Energy we nominate as the bringers of Life. None can conform, none can out-perform the Greater Energy, that which declares for Love. Following the arrival of Love, perceived as the Great Mother emerging from the waves of the Great Ocean, there was the bringing through the emancipation of her son, the One, the founder of Intelligence, who posted the three principles, **Truth**, **Equality**, and **Unity**. None of which is capable of appearance, of expression, without the uniform measure of Love energy emanating from the unseen living foundation.

Great Lucifer: So welcome in this evening. *The small group returns the greeting.* You might wonder who this is that is speaking with you. You might say that I am known as the Greater Energy. I am a voice for the Greater Energy. So I am not a persona and as such I am not an entity.

Through your developing years, which we would count as somewhere in the ten to twelve year mark you have met any amount of entities. You have met any amount of a conglomerate of entities. Some were with you wholeheartedly and some were decidedly against your position.

You are now into the new play. Let me tell you without reserve, that we, the Greater Energy, are calling the shots. Are we a conglomerate? We would go a little bit further than that. We would suggest that we are an aggregate of energies with a combined interest in the further development of the cosmos. A conglomerate is never more than a mix of different patterns, different ideas, or interests.

With us we are not subject to those disparate ideas. We have one driven understanding. We will make our understanding known and available to all those who are prepared to stand still and listen. We are those determined to establish Love throughout the cosmos and its planetary children, those beings of different planets in different star systems.

It is important for you to understand that everything that you had given to you, or promised to you for the last ten years, has no future. Those who made those decisions, those who made those promises, those who wished you well for your future are no longer at the helm of the wheel. The old saying goes, 'if wishes were horses beggars would ride'. There is now a new helmsman at the wheel. So your allegiance has to move across to the Greater Energy.

Who is or are the Greater Energy? Well, you are not going to be told. All that we will tell you is that we are adamant, determined, that Love is going to be demonstrated throughout the cosmos. It is a Love energy that is acceptable to everyone who is in the cosmos. We tell you that everyone on the planet is capable of tapping into the level of Greater Intelligence. We will assist those who are ready and willing in making that happen.

We are supportive of the Christos Energy entering the hearts of every being in the cosmos. We will also back Womanhood to be the reigning factor of wisdom, beauty, style, and grace throughout the cosmos. We will also tell you that we are unidentifiable. You cannot put a name to us.

Jézel: You said the promises were not going to be fulfilled, did you not?

Great Lucifer: What was said was the promises that were made by those who wished you well are no longer valid. It does not mean that we will not strike a fresh deal. We do not wish for you to be deficient of funds to be able to perform on the planet that which is beneficial to progressing Love and Intelligence. So we are by no means into killing deals. We are saying you are into a new deal.

Jézel: Sure, I understand.

Great Lucifer: All we are saying is that we and you are not bound forthwith. We do not have a binding deal. You are in a new play. If you like, there is a new producer. The production of the play is taken out of the hands of the Divine Mother.

You may well have some idea who the coordinators of the Greater Energy is or are because you have had a sample of the Unnamed, Los Diabolos, the Lords of lightning, the energy…though you are not familiar with the energy…that is behind the Great Dragon. Did you think that the Great Dragon was the end of the line? Did any of you consider that the Great Dragon is no more than a visage…what is the word we use for the entity?

Satania: Hologram?

Great Lucifer: Have you considered the depth of the Dragon Energy that which seats behind the entity? It is a fact that they have their images in the star systems or in the planet…they are projections. The Great Dragon does not answer to the image, or, if you prefer, the projection, or even the mirror. It is the same with you people. I will call you people in this room. It is the same for you. Do you consider that you, the visage, the image, the mirrored reflection, that in effect is as much as you are?

When the Angels asked you who you were, they were making the distinction between what you were displaying and in essence who you are. They did not consider it necessary to bombard you with an idea to create an understanding of where you came from. So they left you teetering on a precipice. And because you teetered you did not have the capability of being able to fathom your own depth. Who is it that speaks with you this evening? Is it someone, from somewhere in your past you know? Is it someone forecast into your future that you would like to know?

Jézel: Yes.

Great Lucifer: The one who speaks on behalf of the Greater Energy will be shown and known as the Great Lucifer.

Jézel: Was it you who came in the other day and cried or at least allowed the body to cry?

Great Lucifer: The Great Lucifer is one who…to the mortification of some of his closest friends…can cry at the drop of a hat. *Satania and Lucifer laugh.* So are there any questions? Doubts?

Jézel: Can you talk about the…illness if you want to call it that?

Great Lucifer: It is not an illness.

Jézel: Well, sure. I just can't think of a word for it.

Great Lucifer: The word for it is simply this: your systems have to be rearranged or re-formed into a cosmic capsule. To do that you have to break apart the old capsule and in a space of forming into the new capsule you are subject to virus attacks. So you have to move through that area before you can consolidate into a new cosmic capsule. It is no big deal. It is a week, a fortnight, three weeks.

So okay, it is necessary to feel some of the same energy as those who are around me. Questions? If you want to move you have to learn to put your questions, whether they are doubts or fears, or whether they are inquisitive of where you will be in the future, you are to bring them up. You have to make them items for discussion. *Pause.* We are without fears obviously. We don't have any doubts?

Satania: I don't see how the people are going to, you know, go into rapport, when you said they are willing to listen and hear about Love. In all the time I have seen people coming in and they talk with you guys they don't really connect. I don't see how it is going to spread.

Great Lucifer: Love that we speak of is subversive in approach. Love does not attack. Love does not dominate. The energy of Love comes from within. It seeps up through the system of the person.

Satania: We haven't met the people that are going to be affected by it?

Great Lucifer: We haven't met the people either that are going to be applicants for it.

Satania: Yes, that is what I am sort of saying. That and the people we meet they go 'yeah' and then they just go.

Great Lucifer: Yes, they go. What the energies are saying is not that they are going to negate what people have already been infiltrated with, or intrigued by, or whatever you want to call it. What they are saying is they are not bound by it. They can introduce the same material from another direction. They are not caught in the heebie-jeebies of it or the argy-bargy of what has gone down already. They will declare the new level of greater understanding.

Jézel: So with the Great Lucifer coming into the body system of Luxor will that be similar to how it will work for the rest of us?

Great Lucifer: Each of you will make the shift if you haven't already made it. I see this as part of the virus, the suffering at this time. It means that you will have a new coat. But I was seeing your old coat like a cockroach anyway.

Satania: Cockroach?

Great Lucifer: You know how a cockroach has an armour coating?

Satania: You talk about a chrysalis type thing, a shedding of the skin type thing. Isn't that what you are saying? All I am saying is the planetary cockroaches don't shed their armour and come out and have another one. Or are we going to come out mutated?

Great Lucifer: No, no. What I am saying is that having had that kind of armour-plate for the human shell that they are to build a new level of…let us say the cockroach with its armour coating is no longer suitable. It is displaced by a cricket. I don't understand it. I don't want to understand it. At this stage if it is necessary for us to understand it then it is going to be shown to us.

But at the moment let's say that the armour plating of the cockroach is going to be displaced and there is a new level of body suit to be fitted that is not armour coated. Are there any more questions? Then Greater Energy wishes you good evening.

The others offer their thanks.

A Second Visit from the Greater Lucifer

Jézel: What is the significance of the ring that you wear on your finger?

Great Lucifer: The ring on the finger at this time simply means that Lucifer has the call on the planet. No more or less than that.

Jézel: Did Lucifer put the sword into the stone to be able to draw it out of the stone?

Great Lucifer: No, no, the sword was driven into the stone at the request of the Mother.

Jézel: And was it at the Mother's request that you take it out?

Great Lucifer: As it was...*Lucifer goes into the feeling of remembrance*...to take the veil away from her face. The Mother energy is Lucifer. Lucifer, if you like, is the transparent image of the male that works on behalf of the Divine and Great Mother. Because they could not go into the perimeters of the planet they required a son/sun to do that work on their behalf. Do not make a distinction between sun and son because they are the same. Sun, if you like, in a planetary term see it as a form of light. So from the great density of the Mother energy they projected a light, which is understood as Lucifer to go into the very furthest depths of darkness to retrieve for them that which had been lost a very long time ago.

And of course the two sons at some stage are meant to unify. In which case then it will be a completion of a diamond state. So we have all these areas in front of us. We have all received our immediate and intermediate roles to play. But don't get fascinated by finance. There are much bigger areas of interest that we are to be involved in regardless of money.

Money will play its part and the Greater Energy acknowledges that we cannot take this world by storm without having the finance to make a mark. They want us at this stage to understand that it is for us an exploration of the intensity of energy; the determination to comprehend our capacity of development, the expansion of understanding, the depth of feeling, and the foundation of Love. These are the areas that we are to involve ourselves in. These are the areas in which we have tasked this small grouping to put their questions, their doubts, their fears, their ideas on the table. It is in this manner they along with us will win the new day.

Discussion with Callers of the Shots

13th December 2012

Lucifer: Lucifer, Jésu, and their cohorts do not come onto planet Earth without purpose. Who is it that drives that purpose? They can be none other than those who have the hand on the cosmic wheel of destiny It is those who take turns at spinning the wheel. It is those who are responsible for executing the Divine Plan and the future planning arrangement...

Let us nominate them as the shot-callers. And Lucifer, Jésu, and cohorts are responsive to their call. We obey a greater instinct that delivers Life as it is meant to be absorbed and led apace. Who are we or who are they? We are one.

The representative of the callers moves into the Lucifer body system to continue the discussion.

Rep: Like the Great Mother we do not have self. Those who carry self cannot help but in some way become selfish. So we dispensed with that area some time ago. Selflessness still carries the tinge of self. So we took the word out of the equation. Our interest is in formulating a plan that will promote all things into returning to a harmonious whole with a capital W. The big W.

The wheel spins, but we are not gamblers. We do not put our chips on the table. And why, simply because we run the game and the house does not bet against the house. We can tell you that those who want to bet their chips, which means their money against the house, cannot possibly hope to win. It is a lesson though certain entities that are cosmic and even beyond cosmic fields have still not realised because in their selfish indulgences they still think they can carry the day. Ah, but what about the night?

You may well win the day, but can you carry that through the night? We say, 'no way, Jose'! The night is guaranteed to replace the day. The night initially was the darkness that preceded light. It gave over its position so light could have its play. When the play is done and the curtains are drawn then night once more takes...again there is no word for it. Some people call it the void...

Satania: Space?

Rep: If you like, empty space. There is to be in a biblical sense the gnashing of teeth. For those who want to take a bite out of the night find they do not have a tooth-hold. So when you bite and you cannot fasten on the moment then the teeth gnash together.

So we gave religions their opportunity to perform to the best of their advantage and they could not. It was not from the want of trying, for what has been said by our protégé, Lucifer, trying has never ever succeeded. Once they got involved in trying they became extremely trying. Had we been in the self, no doubt we would have wanted to have crushed them like cockroaches a long time ago, but our tolerance is expansive, so we would prefer that religions destruct themselves. They do not need any support to make that happen.

Let us move on to science. Where does science derive the idea that this planetary orb is real? Yes, well fairy floss is real, except when you put it into your mouth it melts. And were we to take a bite out of the reality of planet Earth it would also melt because it is not substantial. Never was, never will be, while it is in the third dimension; because the third dimension is an area of illusion.

The planet and its people have to come out of the third dimension to find some level of reality. That is not to say what is composed in the cosmos is real either. It is just that it is more real than planet Earth occupies. So everything that you are able to see, whether you can comprehend it or not, if it is visible in some form to the senses, it is a mock-up. It is the illusion of the magician.

When you reach out to grasp the illusion then you are deluded and you are dumped back onto your own area of dreams. So it does not matter how many times you gird your loins, you pick up your sword, you defy the elements, you cannot proceed against us because all we do is laugh. It is like the child that wants to take on its parents. All the parents will do, if they are tolerant, is laugh.

Jézel: Welcome in. Who is it that is speaking with us this evening?

Rep: You invited us in, or at least Lucifer did. You can call us the callers of the shots. We accepted your invitation. So we are in for a brief period only. Then we will go back to do what we do best, which is the spinning of the wheel. We will say again what has been said so many times, we do not offer you anything. However, if you are competent to ask the questions then we will give you the answer necessary for your next area of development.

Cosmic Energy

Satania: I would like to ask a question about what is real. You said what is here in the third dimension is not real and even in the cosmos is not real, so what area enters into real?

Rep: So the real as seen on the planet and in the cosmos is spelt r.e.e.l. In other words what you are seeing is a roll of film.

Satania: Okay, when is it real? When is it not actually a replay?

Rep: When you are capable of depthing the very base of who you are.

Satania: So you are saying that people on the planet may be in the real because they have depthed.

Rep: No, what people on the planet would have gone into the real?

Satania: I am talking about the body you are talking through and Jézel.

Rep: No, they are still in the roll of film; R.o.l.l or r.o.l.e if you wish. They are still involved because you see the people you are speaking about on the planet are not who they are; they are projections of who they are.

Satania: Yes, and that is why I asked what area would there be when it is r.e.a.l.

Rep: When they move back into the composite form from where they have been projected.

Satania: And how far back would that be? Is that going back to the Great Ocean or is there still realness outside of that Great Ocean?

Rep: Let me say that you can experience that realness even in your situation today, but it will only be glimpses.

Satania: Okay, the body that you are talking through always says he is not on the planet. To me that means he is already on the fifth dimension and that is when he is into an area of realness.

Rep: The realness that you speak of is a tenuous line that exists between this character that you mention and our selves. While that line is open or connected then he has realness.

Satania: Is it always going to be that fleeting while on the planet Earth?

Rep: While we are speaking of planet Earth as it is today, yes, but then it moves, which means it takes a closer step to Home. Then of course the line strengthens.

Satania: What stops that being more so than at this present time? Because of the density of the atmosphere, is that it? It is not the connection.

Rep: The denseness of the atmosphere has a lot to do with it. However, it is as I stated: the tenuous extension that was necessary to put these people into the denseness. So what I am saying is that is a fine line.

Satania: But is that not into atmosphere? The tenuous extension meaning that has been put out to this third dimensional atmosphere?

Rep: Yes, but what I am attempting to say to you is…if you can take it on…that because the line is so fine there are…I won't call them elements…but let's say interfering areas that are capable at different times to break the line…

Satania: I am not quite sure what line you are talking about.

Jézel: Is that the line the deep-sea diver connects with…?

Rep: No, let us see it simply as a telephone line.

Satania: Yes, the connection back from where you come from. And because of the third dimensional area that line is fragile?

Rep: Yes. It is capable of being broken at different times by entities/energies that have a dislike for our future proceedings. You have to understand this: that we are operating from an area that has the interest of shifting the planet and the people initially back into the cosmos. We are not the only entity/energies that are operating in the greater scheme and they have their own vested interest. They have had the ground coverage for a long time and they are not about to just walk away and say, 'thanks for the memories'. They are intent on fighting for their ground.

Satania: I understand, but I am just trying to work it out in my head with when the planet shifts into the fifth dimension it is going to be a physical shifting of the area as well as mentally, and then there won't be that attack of breaking the line.

Rep: We cannot guarantee that.

Satania: But it will be a physical shift as well?

Rep: You see what you talk about as a physical shift is no more than an extension of the mental shift.

Satania: Okay, so the planet isn't physically shifting then?

Rep: Never was, never will be.

Satania: Okay, but the wobble is shifting. The axis is shifting. So I am thinking that the actual planet will shift like in the actual atmosphere as well.

Rep: Again you have to see that it is like a movie reel. The directors and the producers and the other people who are responsible for putting this movie together are capable of saying 'this part doesn't work so we will cut that', so that eventually what is going to be processed becomes a flowing presentation.

We meet these areas who are disgruntled because their pad is being trodden on by those they have not invited and they are reacting. So then if we can't walk across their pad then we have to go around their pad. That is a diversion. It has not all been plain sailing.

You just do not get into this boat, if we can use that analogy, and pick your focal point of where you are going to go and sail in a direct line to that point. It doesn't happen. We have got to tack. We have got to shift with the tide. We have to run with the wind. We are to do all of these kinds of things, but we will prevail. We will make that point of landing.

Satania: Okay, so Lucifer invited you to come through. Was that to talk about the shift of what is happening on the planet and those who are opposing the shift?

Rep: Oh, the opposers have names. Council of Nine, the Jewry, to a lesser degree the Illuminati, the east coast pirates of the United States of America...

Satania: Is there a team of energies working to break down those areas.

Rep: We have been doing it for quite some time. And we will succeed.

Jézel: What is your relationship with the Great Mother?

Rep: Mmm, now that makes me smile. It is not my relationship; it is our relationship. Because I tell you we are not a single entity.

Jézel: Yes, I understand.

Rep: We will ensure that the Great Mother wins through so that her bountiful area of Love will embrace the cosmic fields. As to our relationship with the Great Mother, I am not sure that we have one. Let us just say that she and her work is on our...what would you call it...table?

Satania: Agenda?

Rep: Agenda, yes, but it is like a table where you lay out a plan and then you work to make sure that the different areas of the plan work as in harmony or...

Jézel: Cohesion.

Rep: Cohesion, yes. So the Great Mother and the Love energy that she is to bring through into the cosmos is part of our plan. And we call that the Divine Plan, but we can assure you that the Divine Plan is still only a portion of the Greater Plan.

Jézel: So you are talking with children of the Great Mother this evening. Are there others that you talk with on the planet who are involved in forwarding the plan?

Rep: We wish. *Laughing.*

Jézel: We would wish also. *Both are into laughing.*

Rep: How nice it would be, to use your colloquialisms, if we could have something like 20, 30 40, 50 selves operative on the planet. I can say to you at this stage you are a very lonely outpost.

Jézel: Surely not a petunia in an onion patch? *Laughing.*

Rep: Well, which could well be. You are the only ones in our senses that smell sweet. There are many who would like to think that they have a grasp of greater understanding, but they fall short of the target.

Jézel: Like those who are inspirational, who are poets, who see a different world, but cannot quite grasp or understand it?

Rep: That was a time when the beauty of poetry was able to bloom in strength. Flowers have a time of blooming and then there is to be brought through a new form of plant life. That new plant life we are nominating is still in a hothouse situation. You must remember that planet Earth and its creatures and its plant life and everything else at one time were in a hothouse situation in the cosmos proper. So that hothouse, if you like, is once more being prepared to coincide with the shift. The children that you see today are carrying the seeds of that future plant life.

Jézel: Yes, I can see that they are a different breed to those who have come through earlier.

Rep: We would like to thank both of you for your attention.

Satania: Thank you.

Rep: You are most welcome. And we would also like to say to you that you are in your essence most beautiful. We would still prefer to remain known only as 'those who call the shots'.

Discussion with Illustrious Ones

12th August 2013

Lucifer was advised the previous day that we should prepare ourselves for a summary of events to be recounted at ten am this morning. Accordingly, we gather, Jézel, Satania, D'Taan, and Lucifer, to meditate shortly before the nominated hour, while we wait for whatever contact is to be made. Then words begin to form into the conscious mind state of Lucifer.

Illustrious Ones: We are ready when you are ready. Please switch on the recording system.

Lucifer: So our greetings go out to the Illustrious Ones. And they are responding by saying as far as they can see we are much more illustrated than they are…*laughing*…not unlike painted pictures.

Illustrious Ones: The summary is being shown somewhat like a court scene or situation, where the learned counsel takes some short time out for a collecting of thoughts; composing the scene so that there is a dramatic effect brought into being by silence. Adjusts the clothing, touches the glasses, and opens the final address, which in this case the jurors are to be seen as cosmic people. And who is most fitting to portray the leading legal counsel? The One.

We, the jurors, are being asked to contemplate all the uncovering of evidence that began with the necessity of placing the four figures of the Divine Family into a capsule and delivering it post haste into the Cosmos Proper. Pause. The Cosmos Proper being an area of great importance should have been in order, but had fallen into disarray because the cosmic entities who were calling the shots throughout the cosmos could not hear what was being transmitted, or if they could hear, they were not prepared to listen.

And none can say that they did not have the information available, because with the very energy they were utilising for their benefit there was carried within it the messages of understanding. Pause.

So the greed that was brought on from initial need ignored the warning to heed. Too much speed. Too much haste, allowing the overgrowing weeds to bring through waste, each in their benighted position as was deemed fit to be placed. Overloads of roguery and chicanery stifled the chaste. Out of balance, helter-skelter, spinning round and around. Oh, what a playground!

Now the chickens are to come home to roost. The Eagle soars in flight.

Now the Great Dragon stands vindicated for having shown support and protection to the young Rose in its initial blooming.

Now the Lion has left its mound and is seen to prowl around the ground.

Now the voice of the Great Mother is saying her lost children are redeemed.

From out of the past dream is born a New Day. A schema of being that draws down a fresh play.

The question before the court is to be put for the jurors to consider: who wrote the script for the Divine Plan? Or is the script being written in the very moment? Who holds the pen? Who dictates what, to whom, and where? And why should there be a need for a hand to hold a pen? For if nothing is the author then no one displaying life as a thing can claim a copyright.

So it is that the children are to share the abundance of what is not, nor ever was willed. The term what in use being what is loosely called reality. And nothing in being who is responsive to energy does not lay claim to its workings. So have the children learned that abundance when gifted is not an invitation to a free for all?

That division was never meant to be separation. And even when separation became to be seen as reality it was never meant to inflict excessive pain so as to create enemies. So now in the joy of homecoming it is time to break down the fences or defences. To merge in the understanding that one is a first step that must be taken to rejoin what was initially broken apart, but never wrought asunder.

The hardest part in inviting recall is in reminding each and everyone 'Love is all'. Every potent, every piece of distinguishable reality, is proportional. Like fitting together a jigsaw each is to find its appropriate place. Therein to find grace and in the vaulted sky of night time there you will see the face of the Great Mother etched. Then we who acknowledge ourselves as her children will know our work is done. Our time of venturing forth is over.

One final thing has to be said: when the book is written, on the back cover the circled symbol displaying **Truth**, **Equality**, and **Unity** surrounding the core centre of Love will be demonstrated.

It is the wish of the Great Mother that her children find their way Home through an understanding of that which the symbol portrays.

The One has stated what was always meant to be said. And it is the book that advisedly every lost child will read and in that moment know their true selves and find their way Home.

So for us who sit in the Hollow Arena this morning you might say we are being given another clean slate, wherein our planned or plotted work has already been scribed out for us.

The cutting tools are on their way. You might see the job at hand as a prefab situation where the pieces so crafted will enjoin to create a new cosmic dwelling we are calling the Fifth Dimension.

Discussion with Colour & Sound - 1

13th November 2013

Colour & Sound: It is time for us to now look at our futuristic planning; for the development of Divine Womanhood on behalf of the Great Mother and the accompanying Intelligence on behalf of the One.

Though we may step back at various times because we consider it is not suitable for us to come forward, do not fall into the trap of thinking that we have left the area or we have left off the desire to implement the greater energy of Love.

Who are we that speak? The only way we can demonstrate it is to say that we are a conglomerate of energies that are determined Love and Beauty will be manifested amongst the people on planet Earth. Why planet Earth? Because it is the springboard for the star energies in the cosmos to have the opportunity to dive into their futuristic developed understanding.

Whether they are prepared to like it, or whether they don't, is immaterial. Their intelligence quotient is going to be improved and delivered to them from this tiny speck that has been called planet Earth. And those who will be instrumental in making planet Earth the central focus of cosmic understanding will be the children of the Great Mother. So just because you think at times that you are drifting instead of shifting do not lose the memory of why you have been put here on this infinitesimal planet.

We do not expect you to understand the politics of the Greater Nine. And besides it is not your area anyway. For you to go there and attempt to enquire will simply cause a rebuttal. We repeat it is not your area.

We that speak with you this evening are not locked into the Greater Council. We acknowledge the area of work of the Greater Council, but we are not subject to that council. Then who are we you may well ask. We have no boundaries. We have no limitations.

Jézel: So then you would not be living in any dimension.

Colour & Sound: Without dimension. We fashion sensitivity, but we are not subject to sensitivity. We are capable of demonstrating Beauty. But if you attempt to place a control on Beauty then we disappear. Or, if you prefer, we step back. As for Love we are immersed in that energy. But attempt to touch our fronds and we close the show.

So what is our link with you who sit in this room this evening? We offer you nothing and in return we do not require anything from you, because in every requirement there is a demand. And what you cannot give willingly for the greater good has no value. What you cannot lose agreeably has no worth.

Sometime in the future you will find your designated role or pattern, but you do not have it as yet. And when we say 'sometime in the future', it may be a week, a month, a year, or ten years. If you demand attention you will be denied. If you are submissive we no longer need your service.

Jézel: In what way do you require our services?

Colour & Sound: In a state of equality. The same as we will request that you link and involve yourself with people on the planet in a state of unification and Truth. To mention Truth in this day and age is almost laughable. I am not saying that Truth is laughable. What I am saying is that the idea that humans have of Truth is laughable because their whole living system on the planet has been built on a lie. So how could something that has been demonstrably a lie for so long have the audacity to declare itself as Truth? Truth does not come from the past. And therefore it has no future (drawing energy from the past). Nor is it available in the present.

Jézel: So would you call it ephemeral?

Colour & Sound: No, Truth is solid. Ephemeral is something that arrives and acts and then disappears. Truth is solid.

Jézel: But certainly not evident in third or fourth dimensional.

Colour & Sound: However, it can be experienced in the fifth dimension. So Truth at this stage, if you like, is still a futuristic principle to be endorsed and…I like the word…untangled. Of course, at the end of working with Truth is acceptance. It is enough to know, or have the awareness, that there is the principle of Truth. And acknowledge that it is so. Allow it has its time of future expression and with that in the state of acceptance let Truth embrace you.

Jézel: So do we need to go through the stages of Equality, and Unification prior to embracing Truth?

Colour & Sound: Yes, Equality as far as we understand for the people on the planet is going to be their first task. Through an endorsement of Equality will develop or breed Unification. And when those two areas find a platform or foundation, or whatever you want to call it, then Truth will be available for open discussion. The baring of the soul, if you wish. The remembering of the human birthright. The contemporised understanding of human purpose. That is how we see the flower, which has been called the Rose, unfolding its abundant petals.

Jézel: So the bud goes onto full bloom.

Colour & Sound: And the humans move, along with the planet, into a new phase of future life called the fifth dimension.

Jézel: And with that it strikes a chord throughout the cosmos, does it not? Does it not light up the rest of the cosmos into a shift as well?

Colour & Sound: We have stated to you at different times how simplified is the situation. That in a family when a new baby is born everybody has to move their position because the baby has precedence and everybody must step back and acknowledge the new child.

So it will be with planet Earth when those that are in the cosmos see the fantastic beauty of the new born child they will be in awe and they will move accordingly to give the new baby the space it is to occupy.

If you like, planet Earth at this stage is clouded or shrouded in mystery. After all, when the baby is in the womb of the mother nobody knows what its future is likely to be when it is delivered.

Jézel: So earlier I was considering there would be a revealing of the mysteries when Earth moves into the fifth dimension, or you could see it as being born as a child unto the Mother.

Colour & Sound: Actually it is being born unto the cosmos. It is the Mothers that deliver it. When I say born unto the cosmos it is born into the family. It is the Great Mother who gives birth.

Jézel: Yes. What I was saying is it becomes part of the family of the Great Mother...if that is the right phrasing...

Colour & Sound: And I am not sure either because there are those who do not agree that they are family. There is still some of that mind. Be that as it may the Divine Plan is symbolically placed to carry through the features that we have spoken of.

Jézel: So you have spoken with us before, but have you spoken with us as a conglomerate, as you were saying?

Colour & Sound: No, we have come through in individual form, but now we have gathered strength and so it is more appropriate to nominate us as a conglomerate of energy, which is not subject to past enterprise.

Jézel: Or time and space for that matter.

Colour & Sound: We are of the New Day. As you were put on the planet to be pioneers so we are set in the cosmos as like pioneers. Then of course when I say that, I am not saying that is where we are coming from. What I am saying is we have been given the opportunity of being positioned in the new form of cosmos.

We have gone as far as we can go this evening. Be assured that we will be in contact regularly. I am just considering as to whether you require us to have some form of name for acknowledgement. Nothing comes to mind but the next time we come through...

Jézel: We will call you nothing then, shall we? *Both laugh.*

Colour & Sound: Yes. Next time when we come through I am sure we will have worked out a code name that is suitable for our identification.

Everyone gives thanks and the entity leaves. Soon afterwards, Lucifer receives an addendum:

Colour & Sound: The entity that speaks this evening represents colour and sound. Our purpose is that the cosmos will become one harmonious area. We are not about bringing the cosmos into alignment and then busting it apart by shooting arrows at each other. The merging into bonding is to be achieved without glue. It is to be consensual.

Cosmic Energy

Discussion with Colour & Sound – 2

30th November 2013

Though we have listed Lucifer as the contributing name in the discourse it is the conglomerate energy of colour and sound that directs the input of discussion for the evening.

Lucifer: The proposition before us to consider is that Intelligence cannot be instigated into circulation unless Love energy is evolved.

Jézel: Yes. It has come out of the experience of greater energies and the cosmos. The greater energies we speak of are those who have utilised Intelligence, and not having allowed Love to incorporate their being, have then lost out. We have had a long hazardous climb to get back into embracing the Love energy with the advance understanding of those greater energies that has filtered through from the cosmic areas. I see it as a great step to not allow Intelligence to feed through such energies unless the Love energy seeds their systems first.

Lucifer: Each of us in this room are au fait with recognising it is the Love energy inside of us that gives us the impetus to involve us in a process of human transition. I am not sure what humans see themselves involved in, but certainly at this stage they are not involved in the understanding of Love energy.

Jézel: They are not particularly involved in Intelligence either I would have said.

Lucifer: Then what are humans involved in? The word being put into my head is modernity. Humans are involved in switching from one area across to another area and the area where they seek uniformity is modernity.

Jézel: However, when it comes down to the base level you will find that their modernity is just another repeat performance; where they are involved in reclaiming and recycling old material.

Lucifer: We need to ask: how is it that people on the planet cannot align with Intelligence? Inside, people carry the Intelligence, but unless you are capable of putting that Intelligence outside of you and then drawing it piecemeal back into you, you cannot be the beneficiary of Intelligence.

D'Taan: Well, I would call that Truth or a portion of Truth.

Jézel: A token splinter, perhaps.

D'Taan: Or a splinter of Truth by projecting Intelligence out and then bringing that back in is an alignment with Truth.

Lucifer: In that respect, my friend, you have the cart before the horse because Truth derives from Intelligence, not the reverse. It has been stated very clearly to us: From the Great Ocean depths came the Great Mother and from the Great Mother was born the One. From the One came Intelligence. From Intelligence came the three principles, **Truth**, **Equality**, and **Unity**. So they are decisive steps and you cannot retract on those steps. So you cannot say that Truth breeds Intelligence.

D'Taan: No, I wasn't. I was saying it was realignment or…

Lucifer: Oh sure, I am okay with what you are saying there. That if you were in effect to involve yourself in Truth then in understanding yourself you will rebuild or perhaps, more suitably, in-build a greater form of Intelligence. You will also do the same thing with **Equality** and **Unity**.

That is if you are prepared to involve yourself in either one of those then you are also going to find that you have in effect developed a greater level of Intelligence. But you also must remember that those three areas have been projected from Intelligence and Intelligence has been projected from Love and Love has been projected from the Great Ocean and in the building of greater understanding we do not need to go further back than that.

Then there are the significators that we work with, such as we nominate the Great Mother as the face of Love energy. That we nominate The One as the face of Intelligence and down through the totem levels, if you like, there is any amount of greater energies. But that doesn't mean that those who are backing us in this work on this planet are necessarily of that line. For instance, the Great Dragon…

He is not in that…certainly not grade. I don't mean to downgrade anyone or anything. What I am saying is in the steps that come down from the One we should not consider that the Great Dragon is in that stepping down because he is not. And where the Eagle, the Lion, the Tiger sit or fit…these are representative of great fields of energy that are beyond the bounds of the cosmos. We are subject to their understanding.

And though the greater energy certainly invite us to match with them in advanced understanding, we do not find that level unless we find within ourselves the simplicity of accord to engage **Truth**, **Equality**, and **Unity**. When we are able to match those forms of understanding within ourselves we are embraced by those giants of elementary understanding responsible for promoting cosmic development.

They invite us to enjoin with them, but that can only happen when we are neither proud nor are we obsequious.

Jézel: I see that we are to burst through the concrete wall of oblivion. The concrete fixtures that are blinding the people who are on this planet are the areas of belief and conditioned opinions. Unless they gather fresh mental strength, which is the energy needed to break through and smash the concrete façade…at this stage planetary people are not able to do that.

We have had the benefit of the greater energy support to enable us to build the strength to make the breakthrough, and also the desire to achieve the breakthrough, which is an important asset, to smash the concreteness of beliefs. So we can then move into the areas of **Truth**, **Equality**, and **Unity,** which again will take us to the next level of cosmic intelligence.

Lucifer: We are placed in particular situations for the benefit of greater learning and understanding. If you can hold your place, if you can take on board what is being offered to you, then in turn you will have a role to play in developing further the greater understanding. If you deny your **self**, which means you refuse to identify with the greater energy, then you will be removed from the board of the greater plan.

It is in the keeping of each of you as to whether you are prepared to continue to take one more progressive step.

Chapter VIII.

Fifth Dimension & New Day

Dawning of the New Day

There cometh a hush, a dreaded pause
When the lion shall unsheathe its claws
The bright-eyed tiger decides to stalk
The tangled ways that humans walk
Church and science will both stand back
Where colour replaces white and black

When Angels engage in circumstance
Humans lose thought in merry dance
Starbursts replace width and length
Female energy regains its strength
The Rainbow Trail sky-wise appears
Dark clouds break, a New Day clears
Give yourself over

Dawning of the New Day

Little do people locked in society realize that it is the energy of soul stirring awake to greet the dawning of the New Day.

Humans have filled their lives with nonsensical chatter because they cannot find acceptance within their proprietary owning of singularity. Their minds are compelled to run amok because they cannot sit still. Extreme noise in society has become preferable to silence in an attempt to allay the emotional pain that overrides peace of mind. There is no peace of mind available for the psyche shell has been shattered and scattered into a mass of pieces that are contained in duality. Peace is only available for those who can resolutely put their separate pieces together.

The rational mind has walled itself into a series of box frames as a protection against envisaged enemies that are deemed to be seen as opposites or opposing forces. The defensive mind can no longer hear or see anything that does not agree with its falsified patterns of belief. The walls of the ego driven mind are bereft of relief without windows and doors. For many people the semi-conscious lives they lead are dark and bleak with no obvious future in sight. The diminished light that is cast in society is artificially weak and produces huge shadows. Thus human minds because of their ego frailty are afraid of their own shadows.

These reflected shadows forming from painful memories have filtered down through their planetary lineage. The memories holding the unresolved issues are indicative in the psyche and are distributed generically through DNA strains. The glug of contaminated issues from the past are retained and maintained in the blood stream. They are a debilitating force and over time weaken determination in resolving areas of human malcontent. It is high time they were removed from exerting undue influence on human systems.

Can humans deny the past fashioned by their forebears? Not any longer. The past is about to catch up, overwhelm, and meet with future events. This world people occupy is being catapulted into another dimensional space that is called the fifth dimension. Can you remember being somewhere like there before?

It is so beautiful. Some people call it the doorway to Home. The colours are extraordinary. The music carries melody that no longer jars the nervous energy held captive in psychic disorder. The innate ability to smell and taste is restored to their correct levels. Touch is mandatory and goes with the new found territory.

The rational mind gives over to advanced forms of understanding and telepathy once more becomes a regular tool of communication. Power and will are converted into rhythmic movements that lighten the loads of endeavour. Grace and beauty are appreciated and children are born with accelerated wisdom as part of their birthright. Truth appears and is accepted without the present day necessity to garnish our daily lives with petty lies.

We who are requested to foretell of the planetary shift to come are not dreamers. We are messengers. Our visions for the future that we are required to share are planted within us. Yours are also there within the source of being. Learn to sit still and locate balance. Then the doors to the Cosmic Mind will open. Let go of haphazard beliefs that hamper the natural flow of human mind development. Then the windows of the soul will also fly open.

Most of these happenings will occur gradually over the next ten years. No longer is there to be the malady of the sickened soul that yearns for a return to a dreamy yesterday. The melody of the New Day is upon us. The pioneers of cosmic joy are busy clearing away the musty cobwebs of yesteryear, which detail becomes apparent and dismissed in the light of expanded consciousness.

When will you agree to enjoin with others in sharing a new cosmic rearrangement to advance communal benefit? To progress into states of living free what should you be prepared to do? The first step we ask of you is to undo what is no longer necessary to hoard. Let go of the restrictive ties from yesteryear that bind your planetary mind. Protection, the social uniform of the oppressive ego, is passé. Sit still and consider. Is it not time to start spring cleaning the wasted cobwebs out of your psyche? What will you lose except the socially impaired mental diseases and body pain that suggestive medicinal cures have force fed into your system? What will you stand to gain by losing or letting go of past impediments?

There is a new day of balanced order arriving post haste. The Angel choirs are singing of the incoming essence. The Divine Family awaits your return to Home. To hasten your footsteps the Divine Mother and Father have sent their two sons, Jesus and Lucifer, to meet with you. Be available to greet them without the rancour of past grievances. Life in the New Day is assured with an awakening new mind embracing cosmic awareness.

Recovery and Discovery

Long ago, three million years almost in linear time, humans were deliberately cast out from their incubated state onto a road of external discovery. Now the turn around, which is recovery, is set firmly into mobile space and will inevitably take place. The cosmic spotlight is firmly trained on planet Earth and its people as they are moved into position to access the Fifth Dimension and beyond greater understanding. Now is the time for the uncovering of old secrets.

Who wants to know of their past heritage and purposefully ordained future? Of the cosmic strains of colour that are to influence their lives? Who are so far out and disconnected that they will reject the opportunity to review their immediate programs so corrections can be made where necessary in assisting them to withstand the heat of the planetary shift?

The ego protection cover over mind is like a plastic sheet built and maintained by a falsity of patterned beliefs. It is advisable to remove the fabrication before they become subjected to the flaming torch of Intelligence that heralds in the oncoming New Mind.

Humans are like caged prisoners, each locked away in their own singular type mind cells, devouring whatever they are fed each day from the sensory pulp of illusionary media practice. They have long since forgotten the terms of the sentence they were given, or how much time they have endured in recompense. They gaze through barred windows into mental quadrangles of artificial light and think because of the bars that it must be the way out.

They have focussed, and still are fascinated by the artificial light of professional knowledge, corrupt though it is in thought assessment. They do not consider turning their heads to see whether the door behind them is unlocked. Who is ready to put their weight on the enclosed door and see if it will spring ajar? Were they to do so they would see the door invites them to walk free into new stages of life and living free.

When people were first locked away they could not accept their situation. Their fear kept them powerless so any efforts to escape were futile and they soon tired of considering forms of release.

Now the messengers, sent to Earth by the cosmic family, walk the land and clearly state, 'Humans have more than paid the overbearing price. For you the darkness of the old ways is over and finished. The veil that denied the dawn of human awakening has been lifted.' Is there a cost attached to the message? The look of joy will be more than enough when people push open the closed doors on their minds and feel the early morning light of the New Day shining brightly on their faces.

Shift to the 5th Dimension

Cosmic Seer's take on the movement into the Fifth Dimension

Date

Q: How would you describe the Fifth Dimension?

Unnamed: It is an arena of consciousness that first bridges the existing gaps in the duality of planetary existence. It removes the disruptions of separation, exploitation, power, greed, and other controlling systems of domination, which have been the order of the day in the third dimensional derangement.

Those areas of derangement humans still carry will not be available in the Fifth Dimension. The Fifth is more about the continuing journey homewards. It is about developing a benefit of communal welfare that is made available to all. There is to be a new form of living free from superficial conditioning; thus connecting the minds of people on the planet with a greater understanding of who they are and their subliminal links within the Cosmic Family.

Q: How does the planet shift into the Fifth Dimension work for each person?

Unnamed: The questions facing the global populations of planet Earth today are simple enough in theory. Who amongst the populace are suitably prepared for what is soon to eventuate as a reworking of human purpose proposed in a living free arrangement? The prophesied shift in dimensional awareness can be described as defining a climactic rearrangement of human consciousness referenced as an awakening.

The preparation for rearrangement is to come from within the mental apparatus of each person willingly subscribing to the state of living free. The movement can be described as an individual process in cleansing and clearing out waste material from redundant memory cells. We call it on a planetary level the rewinding of the mind when viewed as a clockwork type rearrangement of diffident patterns. It can also be described as realigning with an upgraded rewiring of the old brain system.

Q: Is there to be a merging of the dimensions and what does that mean for humans?

The merging of Third and Fourth dimensions into the Fifth dimension:

Unnamed: Visualize a ballroom that is compartmentalized by two concertina walls dividing the area or space into three sections. Thus each area considers it has its own autonomy where it can do its own thing. There is an exchange system in place where areas can be accessed between the third and the fourth and occasionally the fifth, but to do that one must step outside one room and enter another via means such as a corridor. This method was used for visiting purposes only, short lived, and until now the return was mandatory.

The day will come when the Angels will push a button and those concertina walls will be opened and will effectively reveal the full extent of the ballroom. Thus there is a merging of the third and the fourth areas into the fifth and with that movement all three compartments become one. There is just going to be one enlarged room and your mind will be enclosed in the fifth dimension. That is how it is going to happen.

The problem for those who would like to have start on other people is that they are going to say, 'What, are you going to allow the people who are dumbfucks in the third dimension have access into the fifth dimension without them having to do the hard yards?' The simple answer is yes, because we did not come on to the planet to be superior to those who are seen as dumbfucks. We may call them dumbfucks and that is okay and we can call other superior ones fuckwits and that is okay as far as it goes. The basis of what we are doing is to make damn sure that everyone, regardless of their attitude, is going to move into the fifth dimension. Everyone!

Fifth Dimension Discourse

Lucifer: People on planet Earth are entering the fourth and final stage of reducing somnolence for the purpose of exiting the third into the Fifth Dimension.

The first stage is to remove belief. Belief, where the projected ego mind is hard at work shoring up fragmented platforms, takes the mental system out of balance.

The second stage is the acceptance of knowing without thinking. Knowing, forming a middle ground of certainty brings the vacuous mind back into balance.

The third stage is developing a greater understanding of life and purposefully living free. Greater Understanding takes the enquiring mind further down to explore the deeper wells of psyche.

The fourth stage is immersion into a temporary deep sleep, a hypnotic term used for entering the rational mind and into the realms of unconscious memory. Immersion is the provisional cradle of Love's waters, a laving experience in the womb that rocks the symbiotic system gently into a relaxing sleep.

Spiritual Development

The Spiritual Development of the Human Species

Building of Awareness featuring an Awakening of Human Spirit

In the opening stages of the new state of spiritual awareness called the Fifth Dimension there is featured a growth of greater understanding informing both human mind and memory. People may think that spirituality is a fixed state in mind relying on locked down beliefs, but like all things that are part of a learning process whatever comes into the everyday mind of humans is subject to rearrangement. So for centuries people have seen religion as a spiritual scion, but like everything that appears to be firm or irreplaceable still there exits beneath layers of human consciousness an eternal movement at work intent on developing an even greater scope for awareness in awakening mind and memory.

Gospel of Thomas: *A reputed Jesus quote:* No one can make a silk purse out of a sow's ear, nor can they drink fresh water from a contaminated well.

Knowledge gained from educated sources of planetary format maintains its share of contaminated water. Education in its varied portions of trained ethos relays sordid information drawn from any number of contaminated wells of past misadventures.

Who is the essential thou or you. It is not a question of enquiry; it is a creditable statement as the mysterious 'who' is in the process of making itself self-evident. In other words spirit energy is becoming more pronounced in daily circumstances. So the importance of brain draining is to clear out the extraneous rubbish that has accumulated over any number of life times. It is not only your life time on notice, but also the lifetime of your parents and the lifetime of their parents and associated friends and teachers in previous societies that haunt the present day.

The Hollow Arena

Never in the modern history of humankind has there been a phenomenon of such an advanced level that is being demonstrated through a woman called Jézel and supported mentally by a reclusive man of letters nominated as Luxor. In October 1997 she was utilized by cosmic energies to make a vocal connection between the galactic area we call the Cosmos Proper and a certain local residency situated on the Gold Coast, Queensland, Australia.

Initially the work involved was concentrated on building an energy base that could withstand the pressure of controlling and corrupt influences on the planet by fourth dimensional creatures whose selfish interests lay in subverting and destroying the beneficial connection being made between the divine and profane.

With the assistance of Angels working in the cosmic fields we established an energy base linking Love and Intelligence into the minds and hearts of many people situated on planet Earth. So regardless of the divisive efforts of fourth dimensional creatures the Greater Energy at cosmic work established a communicative field, an operative area of astral connection that carries the title **Hollow Arena**.

It has a number of brilliant purposes, some that have been realised and other areas that are only now being uncovered. It acts as a receiver of relevant information providing communication with greater entity/energies and Angels that advise us in our planetary progression. It also acts as a transportation station for returning entity/energies that no longer assume influence over local circumstances. So we assist their return to cosmic areas from whence they initially arrived.

Now the cosmic attention is directed to the development of human understanding and the necessary raising of collective consciousness. What has been sold to people as prior knowledge regarding human development is in the main inaccurate. Why is that so? A state of duality invoking a splitting of memory was built from a series of platforms framed in the ego status of minds that separated thought from wholeness.

Nowhere in a planetary recall of yesterday was there a connecting link forming from the foundation of Love energy.

The hollowness that we reference in the hollow arena on a planetary level cannot be measured and therefore to be seen as nothing. Yet on a cosmic level it has a platform of substance. It maintains a descriptive difference between two worlds.

Though we positioned on the planet are cosmic pioneers we could also be classed as swamp removalists. It is from this position we have sent back many entities to their respective beginnings after a short discussion on their contributions to events on the planet, some of which we have recorded by video and audiotape. We have spent more than 17 years dispatching Archangels, Melchizadeks, Ascended Masters, and many other notorious characters, charming or otherwise, back to their cosmic beginnings.

These behind the scene players who took their places on the human stage of life were invited to discuss their past involvements where there were any number of infringements and the parts they played in such. One by one they came in as star energies, planetary leaders, and agents of the fourth dimensional Council of Nine, gods and devils of the netherworld, to lay down their arms and present their selves into the Hollow Arena. Here they stated their case, acknowledged the divinity of the Mother energy, and were then given their release to depart as part of a termination of worldly interference.

We who man this Hollow Arena outpost on the planet are children of the Great Mother. When we speak of the 37 we are referencing the lost children who were instrumental in providing the impetus to put the first species of humans literally on their feet. We, situated in this small enclave, are a doorway to relocating memories from the past. Plus we are assisting in providing an opening to a golden future where a New Day awaits those who will disengage from old habits and release their minds from the pressure of pain and fear being felt by humans in these unsettled present-day circumstances.

A Sitting in the Hollow Arena

Lucifer: It would suit all of us best if we argued less and discussed more. This is not about us projecting energy for our own benefit; this is about us sharing with others the benefit in the greater understanding. What we convey is relevant for all areas of cosmic influence.

Satania: You said at the table tonight that we should be more challenging in discussion. What we were doing before, was that challenging or arguing?

Lucifer: What is it that you are into challenging? Is it someone else's ego that narks and niggles or a demonstration of building your own worth? I am not into quibbling nor am I for argument. What I am asking is whether in these group discussions we can bring into alignment that which is missing in the cosmic areas. We know only too damn well what has gone missing on this planet, don't we? Take a look at it. We are missing both wisdom and beauty. People are missing out badly on understanding Love energy. Intelligence is also being held back so we are missing attributes of style and grace.

Jézel: All the essentials.

Night message received by Luxor and translated: We are entitled to reference ourselves as savants and our network as a medium for cosmic Intelligence. No **thing**, cosmic or otherwise situated, has the power to stop the movement of Greater Energy from delivering on its predictions and promises, as revealed to us who man the Hollow Arena.

Lucifer: I tell you clearly that the energies wishing to communicate will not have a bar of us if we are going to respond to their overtures with displays of selfish ego. We have to be prepared to listen. You have to be prepared to take on board what it is that they advise you. Do not fall into the gaffe of saying, 'excuse me, Greater Energy, you don't live on the planet. You don't have to go to work at seven o'clock in the morning as I do'. If you bring that attitude to the table with the Greater Energy then they will toss you.

Lucifer works to bring the greater energy flow into the Hollow Arena. To do that what he offers to our beyond cosmic trainers is respect. He wants to hear their level of greater understanding. He wants to be trained into measures of cosmic understanding that he does not know. He is not about telling them how wonderful it is being a resident on planet Earth locked up in restraints of Covid virus.

Prior to the merging of certain members in the Greater Council of Nine

Lucifer speaks on the necessity of the Lords of Lightning, Los Diabolos, Shining Ones and others, stepping into the light and making contact and reaching agreement with the Great Mother. Otherwise the families they represent will remain in territorial waters and will not achieve the required statehood necessary for cosmic advancement.

It is important that they state their position, their background, what specialities they bring to the table, and how they see their contributions prevailing to establish a proper order of precedence in the New Day.

So these are the situations that are to be considered when you suggest that the old ways are not to be tampered with. Pride will not usher through a new level of Intelligence. Arrogance has no place in the development of a New Mind. Tyranny and piracy will be seen as wasted efforts by those who are assembling for entry into the Fifth Dimension.

Some may well scoff and laugh and say that we on the planet are only talking about human creatures and when did they ever have the opportunity to be on a level with your cosmic cardiology.

The worm is turning and those who had the upper hand for eons are about to be taken down and fully immersed in the deeper waters below, an action that will effectively destroy the ravenous leeches and ticks that have fed for eons off the bountiful states. It is impossible to say or name the states as they stretch from planet to star systems, and even in some cases beyond the star systems.

The future is not a singular conformity for hoarding ongoing human ideas. A New Day that is already active means that human life will open to greet a brilliance that cannot be confined. These matters of greater understanding cannot be locked down or denied in planetary arguments for too much longer.

Showcase

Disclosures

The Cosmos of itself does not create or fashion life anew. It replicates in various forms that which is initially given to interpret and command by those of greater energy.

Comprehension in the human mind has not yet assimilated the loosened pieces of thought in order to provide suitable terms for mentally embracing wholeness. In other words, the Cosmos was not the beginning of conscious life entertaining and engaging the species of humans. In its present stage of shifting its dimensional base planet Earth is being shown as a cosmic showcase for the delivery of living matter entering into a galactic future.

Redaction – Editing Process

The advances of cosmic intelligence infiltrating human consciousness are areas of greater understanding we are required to interpret and speak of knowingly. Intelligence cannot be taught or brought about by the candlepower of human will or intentional choice as expressed in scientific research. However, like gold or oil it can be abstracted from hidden psychic reserves in mind and memory through a mix of willingness to learn anew and an alluring enticement of interest in cosmic discovery.

7th July 2020

Unnamed: We can understand why they created the planet and its people because it was intended to be a futuristic showcase for the development of other planets and star systems. Like a young baby coming into a family, the consciousness of the new baby would be reflected in the energies of the older members of the family, which in this case would be other star systems.

The building of the human species is what can be called an enigma. At this stage we cannot see clearly the full purpose in the human species. We cannot see the relationship between humans and other star systems. If you look at human situations on this planet all they seem to do is argue, quarrel, and fight for superiority.

Satania: Then that makes me feel like do we really understand the purpose of us being here to raise the consciousness of the humans if you don't understand the purpose of them being here in the first place.

Unnamed: Agreed, except we are clear in our area of work. Our pioneering job is to raise the consciousness levels of humans. As you can see by the human level of conscious thought at the moment it leaves a lot to be desired.

Satania: How can you be so for the work when part of you doesn't understand why we are doing it? That has always been my thing, the lack of progress in what we are doing. I don't understand where it is all fitting in. Tonight you have said that you don't understand the purpose of the human beings and yet we are here to raise the consciousness of human beings. That is a big disconnect there somewhere, if we have got the job to do something and you do not know why.

Unnamed: Well, there is an old poetic saying, 'ours is not to question why, ours is but to do or die'.

Satania: Yes, but I like to understand things so it frustrates me at times.

Unnamed: It is for you to understand how and where you are to work.

Satania: But you just said you don't understand the connection of why we are raising consciousness...

Unnamed: I can understand the purpose in raising consciousness in humans. What I don't understand is the connecting of human performance with the rest of the cosmos.

Satania: If you already understand why you have to do it, why can't you understand what is behind it?

Unnamed: Well, we have not really met to link up with too many of the cosmic families yet.

Satania: What are you talking about? Who are they?

Unnamed: People on other star systems.

Satania: We have had a lot of channelling. Who are they then?

Unnamed: They have been top dogs or leaders of other star systems. We haven't run into too many ordinary Joes. The raising of human consciousness will not be achieved by planetary activity. It will have to come through the sense of understanding being.

Satania: What is being?

Unnamed: Being is a form of activity that does not require the pressure of planetary action.

Xan: Being has got to be linked with feeling.

Unnamed: I agree. So for that to happen we have to break open or apart the cloak covering society greed. Remove an urge of acquisitiveness that would have us get involved in wanting to buy property…

Xan: Wanting to get married and have kids pass on stale traditions.

Unnamed: Yes, and not get involved in the disarray of political argument and religious bickering. Then people will say to us, 'well, that doesn't sound like much fun to us.' So we were not sent here onto the planet to promote fun. We are here on the planet to perform certain work areas. The guts of what we are talking about I consider within ourselves we in particular are inconsequential.

Xan: What do you mean?

Unnamed: It means we are not greatly important. Our importance was in opening and grounding the Hollow Arena. Being part of that work you can see as important. But we are now only part of the working load. In opening the Hollow Area we were at the cliff face. So we still have roles to play, but it does not carry the same importance as 20 years ago.

Jézel: And right up to 2015 we still had work to clear the fourth dimensional Council of Nine, touch base with the Greater Council of Nine, take on the Big Boomers…

Unnamed: Introducing the Great Mother energy, welcoming the Beyond the Beyond and We who are beyond Memory. Yes, I think we have played distinctive roles.

Xan: That is you. My work hasn't even started.

Unnamed: That is right. So you were meant to learn from others.

May 2014

Jésu: We are one hundred percent behind your endeavours as they are the path of the plan of the Great Mother, so it is so easy for us to do so. It is so simple.

Lucifer: And it is so simple because we are for the Great Mother.

Jésu: To the Great Mother. *Glasses clink.* There is a huge number of stars who have brought themselves into alignment with the Great Mother Energy. So they shine brightly on planet Earth; because they know that planet Earth is the showcase, the way through that whatever occurs on planet Earth in its awakening, its shift into the fifth dimension, will beneficially affect them as a result.

Many are looking affectionately on this place, on us as we speak right now. But you must understand that it is not a case of hundreds or even thousands, it is a case of millions upon millions of stars. We are involved with creating the shift. As we speak they are moving in the direction of supporting the Great Mother.

As we speak there is so much emphasis, so much energy created that many stars cannot do anything else but respond to the Great Mother Energy, and give their all to the Great Mother Energy. In which case they will certainly be recalibrated, shall we use that word? Re-educated into the energy of the female of the Mother Energy. It is so exciting for me, this work. It is sometimes beyond my ken to give an explanation. Lucifer is much more adept in providing explanations. So we are in the throes of shifting. It might seem to you like it is taking forever. So let me tell you it is happening at an express speed in the cosmic area because their time-frame is different to this time frame.

This time-frame is linear. It is a little different in the cosmos. So I can only say to be patient, be still very patient. The L'Hôte de la Mère is…to me it has to be…it is a foregone conclusion. It is a matter of a frame here and a frame there, and it will occur. Thank you.

October 2015

Jésu: Grace is a gift that comes from the deeper understanding of the Mother/female energy, which promotes itself or expresses itself on this planet. And Style has been infused with the joyful cells of Beauty, which again presents itself on this planet. So there is a showcase, a presentation, and the planet itself is to be a showcase and they are the attributes as Satania said that will bring that through.

Jésu: Some star systems and planets have already reconnoitred with you and are fully cognisant with the shift. It seems almost inconceivable that there are still those among the rest out there that are not aware of this shift in relation to planet Earth. Keep bringing the discussions back to focus on planet Earth, because it is the showcase.

Jan 2013

Angel: Yes, hello. When the wave of energy starts to shift, it moves very, very quickly. So starting from the eastern shores of America and riding across the waves of the Pacific Ocean means that it reaches Australia very quickly and moves across and around to the rest of the world. The Earth, planet Earth is meant, and has always for a long, long time meant to be a showcase for the new wave of energy sweeping across the plains and the oceans of planet Earth as it is, or has been, across the cosmos and the Divine Estate.

So what happens is it starts in the lower levels of dimension and then moves up. Then having cleared the greater echelons of the Divine Estate it moves back through the cosmos and having cleared that area once more it is sweeping planet Earth. And that is what we speak of now, sweeping planet Earth.

You can't not be in the swing of things. You cannot have the excuse of work or sickness or otherwise to tell us you are not in the swing. You have had a few dark, ponderous days of waiting. We do not number them or we do not care, either way. You are here on planet Earth and you are here to fulfil your end of the bargain. So it is no use complaining because we do not have a complaints department. *Lucifer and the Angel laugh.*

Chapter IX.

A Cosmic Mind

A Cosmic Awakening

*People on planet Earth
Wherever you come from
What is stored within you
Is part of a greater ME
You are a portion of the eternal
A written heritage in the stars
That is beyond mind and body
We are here to tell you clearly
Energy within soul cannot die
You may deny this message
You cannot deny your heritage
And most importantly
Connection with the Great Mother*

Introduction

Everybody carries the same sparks of Intelligence regulated in their planetary systems. Everyone! That which stops the flow of newly developed understanding from being circulated is what has been locked down in societies from an overload of certified knowledge called education. Knowledge as presented to the eyes for public viewing only gives people half a picture of life. If you want the other half of the picture, which will put you ahead of the planetary game you are required to dive full length into the formation of greater understanding, which is advanced cosmic material tucked away in deeper cells of psyche memory.

So how are we to open the treasure chest of cosmic memories referenced within the human psyche? When the internal door of mind comes fully ajar and memory from the past is revealed and related amongst other matters there will be a reactive spit coming out fast and furious like a hydraulic hiss from those presumed to be authoritarians on worldly matters.

It will come from those in scientific research and human educators for when the cosmic light comes on and shines brightly then people can see that the purported knowledgeable ones are widely inaccurate or off beam in their privileged assessments of human ascendancy.

The thing is that advanced levels of Intelligence are inside each and everyone. Our role is to tap distant memories awake in mind and then shake them all around until the necessary information gets settled, sorted and activated for human advancement.

True love is a paradoxical contradiction in terms that lacks congruence. What is there within the circled area of appointment carrying an itch that as yet cannot find completion even when scratched continuously?

The miscalculated understandings that allowed the initial falling apart to occur can also be used to bring pieces together to rejoin in the heart of belonging.

The first level is an awareness of constructive consciousness moving into minds becoming awakened. Acknowledgement of receiving heightened information from the brain is the second level. Allowance in developing greater understanding is the third level.

So now we sit and we wait for the fourth level of cosmic consciousness to be revealed. The desire within is to access lost memories and live with an open mind. We are advised that **acceptance** in being is making its way through etheric clouds that are still blocking human realization.

Promoting the New Mind and Brain

A structured New Mind linking freely with the backing of a freshly arranged cosmic brain setting

A developed clarity in mind and memory precedes acuity in brain activity.

First of all to ascertain and secure the functioning of a newly structured mind, we are required to take certain necessary steps to bankrupt and dissolve what is wasted material still stored in old memory banks classified as cells or wells in psyche. By bankrupting we mean that human minds are to let go of their hope-filled dreams, the self beliefs, the unrealized ideas of traditional thinking based on duality logistics. We are to leave our memories of previous life mentally voided as in a state of cosmic nothingness.

Just like a bankruptcy in society where it is shown that someone no longer has financial support to continue operating a business; so the same modus operandi can qualify to apply to the old mental systems of thought patterning.

When you can agree that old ideas maintained as beliefs are no longer supportive then you are ready to accept the simple strategy of building a new mind to complement a New Day in the Fifth Dimension. Then the aforementioned articles of planetary dreaming and scheming become redundant.

That which follows closely is a state of nothingness, call it mindless and selflessness, operating for a short period only and then new waves of cosmic procedure, new methods of accruing greater understandings that are worthwhile and effective will start to bring in the light of a new mind awareness.

Recently we were being asked to discuss in a group sitting the Jésu remark that 'Truth will set you Free'. So it is important that we get ourselves involved in grappling with an understanding of the ageless principles nominating Truth as a necessary ingredient in a trinity of human advancement.

To our way of understanding, it links with the process of mentally living free of socially directed impediments. To enter into that reflective zone requires us to first practice the art of neutrality in order to achieve a sense of balance in awakening the everyday mind to appreciate new surroundings. So again, it is a case for inking in a series of visionary exercises called trance-formation, which can arrange for a cosmic doorway to openly lead us unerringly into the Fifth Dimension.

Living free means to operate a new mind without old world recriminations needlessly occupying thought. So again with the clearing out of the old mind mannerisms such as beliefs and conditioned innuendos we are to let go of all accumulated accusations, which are using modern methods of exchange to effectively tie the minds of dislocated people into discordant knots of unrealized future debt.

This old world is entering a new phase of cosmic existence called the Fifth Dimension. One of the significant areas indicative of the shift into a new cosmic terrain will be the upgrading of systems occurring within the human brain and consequentially the alterations of perspective required in promoting a new mind level of management.

So part of the new cosmic arrangement is in improved health in mental restructuring, plus a wealth of greater understanding in that which we are calling the New Mind. The alterations or the rearrangements that are necessary within the brain system and thus flow into the channels of human mind restructuring will appear in the first instance for those unprepared for a rearrangement process as being traumatic. Though, with fresh rearrangements of energy absorbing their tired old systems, people will soon come to realise the benefits accruing in their daily lives, as they enter into a new phase of abundant growth becoming whole in both mind and spirit.

A Well-Kept Mind

Thoughts compiled in a Holiday Setting.

The mind of the everyday containing thought is belt driven by the attachments of localised memory. As time lapses (ageing) so the tension of the belt drive loosens. The problem is exacerbated by the emphasis in society demanding an instant recall of past learning and regular broadcasting of daily events.

The simplest method of reducing slippage in memory is to reduce surplus material stock that is extraneous to where a basic grounding can be established comprising mainly the necessities of clean living and clear thinking.

The mind is similar to any essential workplace area. When the area is kept clean the chance of accident or pest invasion is slight. When the area becomes neglected, just like any untended garden, the weeds will swiftly gain ascendancy. Weeds used in this sense of mind demonstrate an inner turmoil, a disjointed compilation of rubbish-filled doubts fed from beliefs.

A well-kept mind is kept ever flowering with a mental level of gardening skills, a know-how we call greater understanding. In our early days of learning different approaches to problem fixing in mind we were devoid of greater understanding. We did not know any better than follow social patterning. Now the fog of ignorance is lifting and the enquiring minds of children are asking for much more information than society elders can readily supply from depleted stock.

Quote from Shakespeare: 'Let us not to the marriage of true minds admit impediments'. Beliefs are major impediments that mar the beauty of wholeness maintained in memory lodged in the inner self or soul energy. Lack of profound information blocks creditable instruction from being revealed to the enquiring mind. The interrelationship between two selves or two entities when joined as one constitutes a marriage.

Reference Gospel of Thomas: The weeds planted without permission are the beliefs held in memory that are contrary to divine intention and in spreading wildly breed contention.

The opposing areas of humility and pride, trust and hate, faith and heresy, hope and despair, are meant to be brought into balance so they may meld as one and in that joining affair dissension will disappear, no longer to return. Thus, the wayward duality in mind will be immersed back into polarity.

While the stalwarts for societal status maintain their envy of the rich while exploiting and vilifying the poor there cannot be a bed for communal agreement reached amongst ordinary people. So then the polarised efforts of differing areas are to be terminated also.

With the removal of polarity, this third dimensional sphere of magnetized energy is destined to collapse. Then this world and its creatures will determinedly progress to the futuristic Fifth Dimension.

The essence of beauty is bountiful in its transparency. Thus the soul of everyone is beautiful in its transparency.

The dualistic frames, such as hope and despair, are like two buckets that draw their water from the same well. The ego mind compulsively fascinates on one bucket or the other and ignores the content of that which is transported. The water within is the symbol of life giving energy. It is that same energy we nominate as Love.

It has been said that the wish is father to the thought. If it were once meant to be valid, it is not so any longer. It is the Great Mother's wish that fostered thoughtfulness through the birthing of energy known cosmically as The One. It is from his direction and guidance we draw our greater understanding.

Locating the Essential Oil Within

To meet with our future life and greet new standards of living free, each of us is meant to dive and delve deeper within our being. The future for humankind is contained within the hidden depths of greater understanding.

It is for people to realize they do not lack for innate Intelligence. Problems that are maintained in the shadowed portions of the rational mind devalue major areas in brain cells that are meant to be integrated in wholeness, not broken apart into disparate pieces that satisfy momentary satisfaction.

The art of achieving a greater understanding in being is to bring the disparate areas of ego presence into alignment with the essence of soul energy, thus ensuring one combined unit of productive conformity. How are we meant to achieve such a sequence? In this third dimensional state of thinking, it is difficult because the rational mind while still in denial of one whole or true self considers that which is placed on offer for conformity in communal sharing is not seen as sliced bread.

If we are to locate the essential good oil in greater understanding retained within the brain cells then it is necessary to break through the solidified rock formation of mental conditioning that is locked down in reams of generational denial. Educational programs in society training are loaded with continuations of genetic denial. Why, because controlling people are not prepared to admit the generic standards of superior type living standards are built on platforms maintained by a repetitive patterning of obscurities marshalled in manipulative lies.

The secret to learning afresh is to know that the vast expanse of valid memory is still locked away in the depths of the human psyche. There is a secret key within each soul available to unlock that treasure trove of distinctive memories. The art of unlocking is to disregard whatever is presently seen in mind as real and solid to touch. What is believed to be actuality when taken on face value contains much that upon closer examination is shown to be illusionary.

No one lacks for basic intelligence. The problem in society is that the pieces of wholeness in memory are fragmented, disproportionate, and so they need to be collected, connected, and merged back into one purposeful unit. How are we as ordinary people to manage that? First we are to equalize in value the dissident pieces or portions in memory that shirk sensibility.

Mind and memory are caught in a frustrated dual situation demonstrating a recycling process that lacks fruition. When the repetitive mind stultifies from an overload of worthless material the brain cells carrying fresh information cease to cooperate. In other words progression is then caught in a no man's land of cycling and recycling that leads to nowhere.

So to get the fertile brain out of lockdown and activated into automatic gearing that is co-operative requires a resetting of old arrangements into a new mechanism, which we simply describe as the product. The revolving mind is to move past its present dry state of mutated stultification in beliefs to enter into receiving the benefit of good oil, a spiralling effect, producing greener and richer cosmic pastures.

The Product

Living free is to be clear of selfish impositions. Realize that what insincere people load onto the backs of others is mainly excess baggage carried inside the mental framework of diffident selves.

The advancement into the New Day of greater understanding is activated through connecting what is everyday living to link with a Cosmic Mind. The next advanced level of Intelligence growth available for humanity development presently lies dormant inside the brain systems of ordinary or everyday people. At this stage they have not had the opportunity of awakening to connect with the workings of the Divine Plan denoting who they are and what is their hidden purpose when their infinite being was first projected forth into space as a planetary creature.

We have prepared material to demonstrate the cosmic product of vital energy we are offering to share amongst interested people, those willing to advance beyond the constraints of partial knowledge called social education to locate within the intimacy of self-knowing worth.

The product of greater understanding does not discriminate between the achieved education levels of people nor is there an interest in social status. Neither those who have attained lettering behind their names, nor those who have preferred experiencing whatever life offers as their teacher, will receive an advantage of distinctive favour. Within the greater understanding on offer is the opportunity to firmly establish the Product within, which is meaningful in understanding a new Life and the true purpose in living free of distorted planetary conditioning.

The initial information comes in three steps or stages offering waves of fresh mind development: Improved mental health, enriched wealth in greater understanding, and enduring relationships of endearing quality. We discuss various ways to provide substantial strengths of humane capability. The three-in-one package introduces cosmic benefits applicable to advancing communal welfare.

There is a building of a fresh understanding of self-fostering an enduring relationship within each person, which brings added value into home, business, and social activity.

Mind you, if you are to baulk at the simplistic methods we propose for cosmic awakening we are comfortable with using analogy, which suggests an alternative method that is in some way connected or linked psychically. Then you are well advised in using a metaphoric stage coach to achieve the same purpose. Instead of a steering wheel or rudder you have the reins of your future style in living free held firmly in both of your hands. What that means is if you cannot understand what is being stated in the first attempt to realize the benefits on offer then we will find another method of phrasing for you to mentally arrive at the same foregone conclusion.

Three in One

People are meant to meld body, mind, psyche, and spirit into one unified, equalized ordinance that demonstrates Truth without the frills and fanciful touches adorning religious faith and human attempts to harness a science of spiritual denial according to herd-like planetary tastes. We intend to share the realization of living free to confound and then astound any audience under the title of 'Merging Three Aspects of living component energy into one free flowing unit', which signifies wholeness in being.

People may wonder how we can manage to work a human mind and body into sharing equally with an enclave of spirit energy. The simple response is that energy formulated from comic into planetary being can work its way Home in a diversity of styles or fashion. The key to clearing away doubt in the puzzlement of mind is to strip away the façade of planetary thinking that denies Truth in spirit. So let go of a wasted god sense maintaining beliefs and the descriptive phrasing of erroneous ideas waffling on about spirituality.

Truth abounds in minds living free of conditioned impediments. Spirit energy is available for gifted use in any given moment, but cannot be bottled or hoarded for a rainy day. So either use availability of opportunity or lose it as the saying goes. Spirit is beyond description and can only further mystify and mull the minds of those who seek for planetary understandings in zones lacking cosmic awareness.

The immediate role in present day life is to realize we are all involved in sharing a gifted purpose. Some say that sharing is a huge task that still lies further ahead of us. So is the concept of eating an elephant. The mental exercise of clearing brain and memory begins with one bite at a time. Mentally chew thoroughly that which the Angels see fit to put on your plate for daily introspection.

Converting Three Diversities into One

Simplicity is the key to converting three separate segments into one connective energy. First, acknowledge there is presently a separation between linking body, mind, and spirit. Allow for a margin of differences. The body will usually follow the direction of mind so we can allow that procedure to continue. Spirit energy will no longer sit back. So we are to work rejoining spirit with the ego mind sometimes referenced as 'you,' as in the Angel questioning, 'who are you?'

When humans allow even one contingent to get out of sync they are already out of balance. The Greater Energy says the human system is a mechanism. So mentally check in regularly to see which parts of mind and body need attention. Being overheated in mock spirituality, which is not spirit, will take us out of sync. Spirituality in mind, just like religion, is a man-made platform formulating as doctrine. Agreement with all three segments requires an affirmative of neutrality. Our primary purpose is to find the balance within to effectively achieve harmony in enduring relationship.

Where do we begin to reunite? Firstly, we are to strip away the dried out leaves surrounding the flower instead of attempting to gild the lily. In other words, we are to take away extraneous material in mind that is no longer compatible or useful.

Emphasis needs to be taken off the image of body beautiful. Let go of idealistic face sculpture, tattoos, fat shaming, and gym workouts designed to promote a body shape of mean and lean.

The cosmic spotlight is meant to shine on you. So who are you? The ego mind is languishing in the background of its patented work areas. It is not available for comment when the pressure of greater understanding is being applied as a torch of light. When we have dropped off the glamour of body imaging that is a start but we are not yet accessing soul level. So you is the middle game player and it is a new you that needs to take over the steering wheel and weigh into a timely cosmic discussion on moving human parts into a new dimension.

Health Wealth & Relationship

The benefits derived from developing Mind and Memory

Welcome in a balanced study of performance between two areas in the human system that we call presence and essence, which holds the key to building harmonious relationship into every future endeavour that people care to undertake. The secret to building fresh mental growth begins with removing whatever are extraneous material clogging passages in mind and memory that are meant to be cleaned and clear. Such ongoing development then provides for huge increases in mental health, enriched wealth in mind through receiving greater understanding and enduring quality in family and communal relationships.

Improved Health in being: Remove latent areas of pending sickness and accident from interfering in your daily life.

Enriched Wealth in Greater Understanding: Discover richness beyond riches through establishing a process for building new mind settings.

Enduring Relationships of endearing quality: Balanced and lasting mutual relationship within one self that extends to enjoin communally with loved ones and friends.

The Obstacles of Mental Resistance = Beliefs, Duality, Denial, Ownership, Argument

Duality is the persistent fly in the mental ointment. Like who cares to admit they are in two minds when offered choice? A guilt-ridden conscience will always go on the attack rather than concede the futility of its paltry argument for prestige. Blustering words and changing of subject matter are often used as a defence mechanism against realizing there is an opportunity for progress in observing silence.

We are not part of ego evasion and we are not interested in the delaying tactics of senseless argument. What is it that still argues for some small advantage? Is there a part of your system that denies there is unfinished business to settle via reaching agreement? 'An eye for an eye' from the Old Testament teaching still holds a certain vicious sway in polite society. The 'whatever' response says 'okay, I have lost the thread of argument, but I haven't lost the fight'. That would be like dreaming there is a misplaced ownership of whatever it is you are arguing for or about.

What is cosmic denial? It is a refusal to look closely at who you truly are or represent on this planetary stage. The hooded mask goes on instantly whenever the rational mind is questioned on its viability. Who wants to admit liability and reveal the so-called unsavoury portions of each particular persona?

Ego slumming is popular fare in society values today. The ego mind weaves, feints, dodges and ducks the spirited determination required in fateful decision making. It is time for the human system to call a halt to the disdainful mockery of duality occupying as it does the so-called rational mind intent on going nowhere!

To make headway in space for receiving messages of greater understanding we are obliged to clear our minds and memories of superficial nonsense maintained in early belief patterns. Within the accumulation of material we all took on board throughout our growing years, much is valid and carries worth that is steadfast when tested.

Along the way, we also took on what the Angels reference as stories. Simply stated the material the human mind has gathered and stored in its formative years is a mix of credibility and some well camouflaged lies that are not easily opened to the light of scrutiny. The shortcut to attaining greater understanding is therefore made by cleansing the mind of dross maintained in beliefs that we call detritus.

Summary: So the three-in-one package introduces the cosmic benefits applicable to advancing human welfare. That which stands squarely behind the product we offer is the foundation of Love energy. There at the helm or steering wheel to guide human advancement are streamers of Cosmic Intelligence.

Psyche

Consider the word bathysphere. It references the depth of unconscious awareness situated deep within psyche memory.

Let us look at determining a method that can be called a disentanglement of the psyche, which as an initial exercise in clearing and cleansing could be described as a brain drain. The mental problems people suffer from is because there is an entanglement of growth in the psyche, thus the rational mind is wearied from an overdosing of complexity. Why is daily life routine and yet so complex? Because media facilities continue to heap an overload of wasteful junk material they stuff into young and old heads, which are already crammed to overflowing by socially trained measures of formal education.

The psyche is not the foundation of our initial memories. The psyche is a proportional part of an ongoing cosmic journey. When we first managed to break through the psychic boundaries of limitation we were then introduced to entities representing greater energy. Had we not broken through people would still be waiting for a reliable explanation of their cosmic ancestry.

The psyche is like a half way station operating between synchronistic energy and human mentality. The psyche contains any number of unexplored memory banks seated behind the wall of an arrogant ego process that some people mistakenly call the unconscious mind.

Each human system carries four levels of mind. There is the rational self-consciousness, which is ego driven, the subconscious, the unconscious, and the automatic, which is instinctive. The subconscious level seats beneath the self-conscious. So what is the difference between the unconscious and the subconscious? There are contained various memory banks in the unconscious that are proportionally part of understanding the journey homewards.

The well of the subconscious carries fear, as it carries the memory of DNA transfixed pain. The unconscious mind does not. The unconscious is aligned with the internal self or soul energy, whichever name you prefer. Soul energy does not have planetary fear, so it does not experience mental pain. It is the subconscious mind that irritates or aggravates the self-conscious. It carries reminders of unfulfilled memories referenced in the strains and strands of the DNA.

So each human system is still working subconsciously to clear away old patterns that were never completed in other lifetimes. To get resolvement of unfulfilled memories you are to mentally dive. You are to get down and underneath the problem areas, which we call splinters, and splash around, thus compelling them to come to the surface for the light of clearance.

Smashing the Mirrors

This third dimensional world of existence maintains a series of distorted mirrors. They cannot offer humans truth, beauty, and goodness as an objective picture for guidance while mistaken ideas of planetary reality lie in the minds of disturbed observers.

The illusion cast that clouds human perception is called Maya, the false one. It is described as a series of mirrored frameworks that deny sensibility.

Our set task is to smash the mirrors deflecting greater understanding. Find the answers appropriate to elevating advanced forms of communal agreement contained within your psyche. Perfection falls far short of fulfilment. When your cup is filled to overflowing drink the wine supplied no matter how bitter are the dregs.

Love energy is achievable through embracing adversities in life. Do not envy those who seem to make life work seamlessly for they are still asleep and are satisfied with their dreaming states.

Better to become awakened and feel the pain of awareness in knowing than slumber in states of separation.

He, who pretends or affects to know all, knows not. He who takes the time to see the worth in each other will find the same within and therefore be found worthy.

How can we rise out of this sorry mess called civilized society if **me** and **you** do not agree to climb? When the **me** becomes **you** and the you is me then with single mind and heart can we walk out of planetary hell. Hell is an illusionary state made real by pragmatic minds. Remember it is the heat of fire that tempers the steel. That relentlessly burns away the dross and leaves the purity untouched. Submit to the flames of Truth and the passion of duality is no more. Nor was it ever there except when kindled in our dreaming states.

Let this world deny you and you will find Life. Deny the life and you are once more locked into bondage. Accept the world without the boundaries of judgement and then we are free to walk beyond without hindrance. Whenever we train we are conditioned. If it is the body we exert we are muscle bound, no longer supple. If it is the mind we train to achieve, we are once more limited, not subtle. When the spirit is being restricted, orthodoxy is the chains that bind.

Love finds those who are empty of misgivings. Give all things equal value. If we choose to live foolishly in the now the past will sabotage our future. The now lacks a suitable balance between memory and desire.

The opportunity is here to repair old karma; to create wholeness, and expand consciousness by merging different elements of the self.

Memory is a mirror image of past happenings. Problems arise when the mirror is partially obscured. Obscurity forms from denial. We cannot see ourselves as others see us because we are locked in the falsity of mirror imaging. We deny our inner being. The present picture being portrayed as life is no more than a human image of wants and needs fed by the desire to remember a life free from daily encumbrances.

Everyone carries a mirror image of what they are. When the glass is smudged, distorted, and smeared by beliefs and other emotional claptrap it is time for an overhaul by clearing the mind and applying a fresh coat of polish.

A rule of thumb: What we observe as detrimental in others reflects a distortion of what has activated on the inside of our mental framework.

Reflected Glory

Lucifer: I ask myself 'what does it mean to represent reflected glory?' It means that the energy we represent cannot be presented in its true or pure state. The only way it can come through is via reflection, but when it hits a mirror, it is then caught in a mirage of beliefs. So it is important work for us to step up and smash the mirrors demonstrating falsehood.

Realize that the Divine Mother who represents the epitome of Love energy provides a stepping-stone to where the core can find its reflection. What we are saying is that the Divine Mother is not the mirror. Because we are on the planet, it is required of us in our present state to be the mirror. Then our work is to smash the mirror so that the Love energy moves through and further on. How beautiful it is to know we are progressively part of the process of on-flowing Love energy.

The big point in living harmlessly is to stop the arguing within the mind and what is without will dissipate. If somebody has a viewpoint and it is different to yours, it is a waste of time trying to convince them that your understanding is superior to their trained knowledge. It won't happen. We have to concede that people won't necessarily agree with us. We can then decide that argument has no valid purpose. With regard to argument, you need to smash the mirrors of comparison, which means to allow the influence of other personas to move away from you.

The Angels say that the mirrors in play today are reflective of human dreaming states. In smashing the discordant mirrors of beliefs, we destruct the dreams of folly because over eons in time the intended patterns for living free have become distorted and are in mental disarray. There is a requirement to collapse whatever is featured as an outworn past in order for a new mind of greater understanding to be assembled free of psychic entanglements that continue to hamper human growth.

The mirror is the separation between what we call the two selves. If smashing the mirror suggests it brings on seven years bad luck, you can be that lucky that superstition is in freefall. If you had done your seven years back when you were a child, you would not have to worry about it today. So it is never too late to smash the mirror, which is the splitting image of ourselves that you have built with the help from other people's input. It is not yours to hold so let it go.

It is a form of ownership and control that comes from outside of yourself, and no one can ever be completely at peace, satisfied, whatever you want to call it, if they are running on somebody else's fuel. So in smashing the mirrors what is it that happens? The separation between the two selves has been kept apart because of these false images that do not match the reflection, and therefore cannot complete the cycle.

Mirror Visualization

Sit back and close your eyes. Begin by taking three slow deep breaths. Let the yawns come out if they are there. Big deep breaths. Find yourselves sinking back into the chair.

See yourself in front of a lift in a tall building. Press the arrow to go down and see the lift opening up and you are stepping in. You are situated on the seventh floor. You are going to go down into the basement. So press the B for basement and you are going down from the seventh to the sixth to the fifth to the fourth to the third…see the numerals above you on the lift…from the third to the second, from the second to the first, now to the ground floor and now you are going below into the basement.

The lift stops and the door opens and you step out into darkness. Just take a moment now to get your bearings and adjust your eyes to the setting. You know there is something you have to do, so have a look around and see across from you that there is a wall mirror. Go and stand in front of it. Have a look to see what image is there and what is being reflected back to you. Have a look at it for a moment longer. In this visualization, you are able to smash the mirror either with your hands or with a hammer that is conveniently placed there, whatever method you wish to use. You are required to smash the mirror image.

What may happen is another mirror takes its place, and then again you might see another image, whatever is reflecting back and once again smash that mirror. So there may be a series of mirrors. We are going to give you a moment or two to go through a series of mirror smashing, the mirrors displaying images. When there is no longer an image in the mirror, when you see nothing framed in the mirror, then that is the time when the mirror rearranges as a portal. You are no longer being reflected back into the past of painful memories.

So now you can move through that mirror. To step through is the way out. We will just give you another moment or two to experience, to feel what it is like by having stepped through that portal. Again for having done the work give yourself a small gift. So the mind will see the benefits if you allow. Now you are ready to come back into the room in your own time, so feel yourself back in the body.

Chapter X.

Love & Intelligence

Love is All

Love is like a tender shower
As it falls like dawning dew
Love is like a slender flower
As the rose we give to you

Should we seek the past and future
Lessons learnt and lost from view
Still the present hopes we nurture
Love is what we got from you

Birds are calling in the twilights
Stones are snuggling in their beds
Angels softly lighting skylights
Fairies stardust babies' heads

As we wander through our wild wood
We are human, let us fall
Then rebuild the blocks of childhood
Until we learn - Love is all

Awakening into the Light

Why can people not see that there is no argument within? Merely a viewpoint of variance between what has been and that which is yet to come to fruition. Our lives, such as they be, whether planetary, star born or beyond, were preconditioned and directed by energy that long ago called the shots. It drove those shots into particular areas so they could come alive; that they could endorse and enjoy the spirit of living energy.

All of this can be seen as building foundations for accessing cosmic life. However, by initially experiencing consciousness, what travail was then to be revealed? For the lives that we were accepting carried pain. It carried the pressure that developed from moving the stillborn into the state of living. It drove a stake for whatever reason between those of goodness and the recalcitrant.

It caused strife to occur between many who, were they given the opportunity of receiving greater understanding, would never have argued. So life in the first awakening did not embrace joy, rather it drove an awareness of consciousness deeper into chasms of subterranean measures nominated as the void. And in those depths, in that darkness, light was not visible.

Though it might not have been visible, it was still viable. Until there was one who was part of that cave dwelling experience who stated, 'enough of this closure. I will take the light that we guard, and I will bring it amongst those who are asleep and need to be awakened to achieve a true realization of their being'.

Of course that decision made him an outcast. For those who had zealously guarded the secrets had no liking for someone who was prepared to make the light of greater understanding visible to outsiders. And for those who slumbered, they were not that enamoured with being told they were to awaken from their dream states and become alive.

Regardless, the torch bearing the light of awakening was lit, and the eternal flame burned brightly. Then it was carried into the open avenues of awareness for the purpose of future development. The flame still burns as brightly as ever. It is a flame that is called Intelligence. It carries elements of energy that override patented frames of knowledge. It carries within the three principles of **Truth**, **Equality**, and **Unity**. It recognizes its substance is drawn from the foundation of Love.

Having been brought out of the cave, once being freed of enclosure, then it could not be contained any longer. The light shines its energy of knowing into the open hearts of all being as it derives its energy from Love.

We, having been placed on this planet Earth as cosmic pioneers, small as we are in numbers, continue to carry aloft the special light of Intelligence aligning with Love Energy. We will ensure from this small established beacon head on planet Earth a brilliance of light that the Greater Energy will use to circulate its rays throughout the greater cosmos. If you like, consider we who speak with you were never born into human flesh. We are sparks of a greater intelligence that intentionally carries the torch of greater understanding into each and every style of living formation.

Within our **selves** we do not lack, nor do we seek to conquer. As a by-line, we have a vital role to play in assisting human development. On behalf of the Great Mother energy, we will deliver the same accordingly.

Love Intelligence & the Great Ocean

Love is the founding energy of all gifted and given Life. Thus Love is All.

Intelligence supports and fosters new levels of greater understanding.

Love has the innate strength and cosmic flare of energy.

Intelligence has the flair of expression.

A new foundation of Life and Living free begins with an understanding of who you are.

When we speak of Love, foundation, and Intelligence they are not necessarily to be seen as being on the same even keel. Foundation is the basic support for Love energy on the planet. We do not have a description for foundation except to say there is a basic supply of fresh energy available for discovery and recovery. We do have a name for the energy of Love, which means then it operates at a level that has been advanced from foundation.

Likewise, we have descriptive names for Intelligence, which means it also has been advanced from foundation. Foundation as far as we can understand is the Great Ocean and we cannot take it further back. We cannot take our understanding further back than to say we in energy form are coming from the Great Ocean and as such for us it is our foundation.

We can work with Love energy so that means it has been moved to a level outside the depths of the Great Ocean. We can work with Intelligence because it also has been moved outside the Great Ocean.

We see it like a vase where the Great Ocean is the base and then the Love and Intelligence are the outer rims of the vessel. We will tell you it is shaped as a crystal vase. And what stems from within that vase is the symbolic flowered Rose. Love and Intelligence with its foundation base of crystal energy promotes the rose of female energy arriving on the planet.

Explanations on the wholeness of living free in the energy of Love and Intelligence can be made available through a rearrangement of paradoxical terms as they surface into light.

Cosmic Intelligence is a beacon of light for those who have aspirations towards achieving greater understanding through living free. Intelligence is the foundation of human awareness. Intelligence declares for cosmic Truth.

Intelligence is concentrated in the flame as the significator for greater understanding, not in displaying attributes of the torch or its bearer.

As human entities people continually search yet do not find meaning in daily life. Love absorbs us when we are prepared to surrender whatever is not rightly ours to possess. Love is energy without qualification.

We are gifted with the opportunity to represent the Mothers and present their level of wisdom and beauty not only for the people on planet Earth, but to all the cosmic energies with their suppliant children. To put all of this succinctly into one basket the expressive phrase we are advised to use is Love is All. Love is not just the expression of Love, Love is also the foundation of conscious awareness and Love energy ignites the evergreen flame of Intelligence to benefit human progression.

For those who were gifted the ears to listen will come to realize their eyes shall open in advance of others to see the light of a New Day beckoning. What will be revealed in their presence is an inner Intelligence, signified through instinctive knowing, which is drawn forth or abstracted from the essence of Love energy.

The Carpet & its Design

It would be fair to say that in every star level we have corresponded with cosmically, that each and every one of those who played in the dual roles of being a user and abuser, with all the good will in their worlds, have still fallen short of their envisioned targets. There is nothing to be achieved in pointing the finger of scorn at others seen as lesser than. There is nothing to be gained by suggesting that any of the entities who fell short in their proposed aim are culpable because they were never really given the opportunity to understand what was to be their target.

That was because the bull's eye of the target was withheld from every form of specified life. The bull's eye represents as Love and the surrounding circle of Love is Intelligence. There was not one formation that built its platforms on will and power that was capable of being able to identify with the bull's eye or its surrounding circle. Not one.

Love declared in the form of the Great Mother energy has no interest in lying down in favour of human diversity. It has no interest in maintaining a separation from its children and for that reason or purpose, it propagated the spreading of Love energy and has progressed Intelligence. And that bow of Intelligence proceeded to send its arrows of innate understanding into every estranged area of the cosmos. But more specifically it sent its most direct arrows into the Cosmos Proper arena, which gave it the opportunity of directing its intention onward into planet Earth.

And then it sent the children of the Great Mother onto that planet to work with the magic of Love energy; to weave, if you like, a garment of Love where its patterns for goodness would become recognisable in memory. So there is the combination of Love and Intelligence at work in the background of the everyday. Love may well be imaged, if you so wish, as a magic carpet and Intelligence the designs woven into the carpet.

Intelligence

Simplicity in words is our forte in mind, mood, and motion. However, the input of cosmic information when delivered carries an overall impact, which we describe as hard yards of contention. Like the cud-chewing of a cow contemplation requires a sequence of extra digestion to gain a fuller benefit than what can be attained from meditation.

The energy field of intelligence resident within the psyche brain cells is nourished and further expanded from the resound of constant questioning, deliberations built into mind from cosmic responses. Similar to a piano in its stillness will not offer a responsive note unless a key is struck. An awakening of the Cosmic Mind is atonement of past memory engaging with present day circumstances. The outcomes determine developed minds of greater understanding for the benefit of furthering human progression.

Planetary information is demonstrated by the declaration of partial knowledge, which is still in the raw surface state of becoming aware of circumstance by circulated stories defining global experience on surface levels. The conceptual/rational mind functions on a semi-awakened substance of basic consciousness only and has no realized awareness of the separateness denying interaction with the inner self or soul energy.

The energy of soul has been given lip service only by religions with little or no recognition of its vital contribution to the continuance and advancement of mind and memory becoming cosmically realized. However, beneath the raw state of materialistic thinking called consciousness by advocates of science there is already in position provisions made ready for more available information essential for the beneficial advancement of human living standards.

Even deeper still there is more information based on cosmic principles and a greater understanding of human purpose weaving into an expanded schemata of occurrences in a pipeline of past and future memories yet to be revealed.

Intelligence in the form of instinctive knowing we call realization is the foundation for all human memory and mental functioning forthwith. Its areas of work for progression are inside every being and therefore paradoxically outside the boundaries of limited thinking set in the everyday minds of semi-educated humans. Cosmic Intelligence is not subjugated to errant thoughts that confess to icons of ideology, be they set in religious frames or carried in distorted theorems of scientific bent.

On more subtle and deeper levels than the imaginary practices of the rational mind can delve, Intelligence intersperses fresh information into a mottled stream of thoughts from which planetary ideas are formed. An idea is simply a platform for demonstrating an association or combination of thoughts that require some type of physical expression or enactment to

Love & Intelligence

be realized. One of the weaker areas in the conceptual mind structure is a language difficulty delaying the conveyance of an accurate understanding of greater energy, which is proposed to soon turn around the unthinking heads of people on planet Earth.

So part of our intelligence work is to accurately translate that which is being transmitted to us from beyond the cosmic fields to a place of no space where accurate memory recall forms from its base of origin. We are gifted with the ability to interpret incoming information from cosmic sources into appropriate understandings to insert the same into appreciative minds. When related correctly this material provides purpose and worth into featured living standards for an advancement of communal benefits. That pretty well describes what we call greater understanding as it draws and delivers cosmic information from some of the deepest wells of intergalactic Intelligence.

****

Intelligence of beyond human presence maintains a series of hidden formulas located in psyche, which selectively drip-feed advanced portions of fresh information into awakened mind areas, servicing those whose activated brains are suitably disposed to accept new material of greater understanding.

There is a quickening occurring in mind and memory of what was previously a slow release methodology. The drip feed is rapidly becoming a stream of designated information that will be delivered as small dots or iota into different places around this modern day world of temporal existence.

Advanced understandings can be visualized like small charges of dynamite, a series of coordinated patterns set with sequential timing, which will blow open and clear away the conflicting fog covering the miasmic thought patterns demonstrating the fallibility of human egos.

The resultant features will provide a promotion of dimensional proportions offering greater levels of intuitive knowing, such information to be validly used for human progression in communal effort, embracing future benefits for a promised fifth dimensional existence that is on its way to consume the latency locked in human suffrage.

Becoming Mentally Aware

To be able to interact with Intelligence and Love as open energy fields it is necessary that we first shed the outer emotional skin of human scruples held in patterns of belief that wax and wane in disturbed waves of duality type programming.

The singular minds of most humans remain stuck in the ego muck of ideological fantasies demanding various types of iconic worship. Thus there is a requirement to remove the false premises called beliefs, those which are profligate without any stable foundation, seriously lacking in the wholeness of greater energy.

We assure you that when errant scruples leave the mind carrying with them the mangled skeins of past ego lines that are fundamentally flawed and worn carelessly as morals, ethics and virtues, their blighted forms of pretence value will not be missed. They have been an incredible overburden layered upon the inner self since ideas were cosmically introduced onto planet Earth by numbers of interfering star entities.

Within the memory banks of people there are at work agitated forms of disenchantment, which are discharging a certain amount of deep-seated misery via the unrealised threads of DNA pressure echoing a reminder of disasters from past events. Though lost in the mists of planetary forgetfulness the urges they still carry are hard at work breaking down the rational lines of surface thinking of people on the planet. An indication of such instances can be subjectively listed as a corona virus nominated as Covid 19 morphing into a Delta strain presently named Omicron.

The misery thus produced forms from interior pain that is destined to erupt mentally and physically under the pressure of modern day engagement. The region of mental disturbance, an underlying factor of emotional discharging, is neither verifiable nor for that matter accessible by ordinary medical methods of cursory examination in matters relating to the human mind steeped as it is in third dimensional consciousness.

Such various types of suspect hit and miss diagnosing of the human mind lack for a foundation of understanding free of religious superstitions; nor will clarity appear as a result of scientific testing with their amateurish habits of psychological prodding and probing. Such methods cannot process nor understand psychosomatic strains of illness and injury on carried into the human systems through the filtered strands of DNA backlog.

When a portion of this miserable memory state comes to the surface in the localised cavity of mind expression the usual tendency is for the persona to become miserly in appreciation. This mental framing activates a body response that tends to express pain into anger, causing in turn an inner revulsion of self that either ends in sickness or some form of accident, certainly a collapse in mutual relationships unless suitable remedial methods of repairing memory are set into action.

In worst case scenarios, where there is a distinct lack of expression, named as depression, there is no opportunity for a natural release of internal rage to occur thus bringing about acts of self-mutilation in mind and at other times suicidal tendencies.

What can be disseminated from misery of this sort is a form of self-chiselling action, which by turning expression inwards results in a vagueness of behavioural patterns, or what is commonly referenced as regression though we see it more as states of repression. It has also been described in previous times as states of melancholy.

Remove the Cause behind Mental Pressure and Pain

Remove the problematic causes of unease caught in DNA memory systems by reducing the effect of mental pain to more agreeable levels of pressure through using advanced visionary methods we nominate as mind balancing exercises.

Some people talk glibly to others of the bigger pictures in life and their determined urge to get there somehow or in some way. How is a question that rarely gets enough external airing to achieve any act of desired resolution. Invariably the focus on how to get anywhere in a continuous dreaming state is drawn back to a minimal point, which engages a form of mind cycling that compulsively reverts to a partitioned space of some discordance.

This condition is caused by differentiated doubts that bounce around in a recoil action in mind, a tumbling effect, which lacks the stability to stand still and amicably form with other thoughts into a stabilised area of unity. Invariably this variance from initial purpose does not manage to close the gap in the mental cycling and the process of on selling an idea to seal the deal has to start over again. The lack of finalizing is not so much from want of effort, but lack of familiarity in character building produces grand ideas of short selling or corner cutting, which do not go the essential distance necessary for completing the whole package.

In real terms, the mental systems of humans pertaining to knowledge and trained technology per se lack the strength of innate energy necessary to complete the desired closure of recycling. Paradoxically, the closing of a situation is essential to provide the next opening for a fresh wave of potent energy to emerge. The closure of past concerns can be seen as a contraction of energy that creates the impetus for an impulsive leap of spiralling activity into the next level of intelligence appreciation.

Intelligence may be acknowledged as the major quality of resourcefulness, but quantity in thoughtfulness also has a role to play.

Projected intelligence can be represented as a neutral zone offering information existing beyond both knowing and knowledge. Knowledge should not to be confused with intelligence. Nor should instinctive knowing be seen as a result of experience. Intelligence forms from the foundation of Love energy. It is the seedbed from which both knowing and knowledge have sprung into being. Both are dedicated pods of arrangement contained within Intelligence.

To understand more, to become aware of greater areas in understanding, we must train our thought patterns to receive extensive mental pressure without flinching. When reverse pressure is correctly applied to mind it assists in widening the gauge, which leads to broader vision or a wider scope in vision and consequently resolves what indiscriminately has caused imprudent pressure. People could resolve most aggravating problems, were they simply able to absorb pressure in mind were they left alone, but societal activities do not allow this suitable state of affairs to happen very often.

Some people think there are people more or less intelligent than others. Basically, this is not so. Some people who appear as intellectuals have the ability to talk about subjects where they carry influence and essay any number of wayward opinions. Intelligence is a further awakening of developed consciousness emanating from the deeper wells of psyche. That some people are awakening and others still sleep does not give start to any one seen as a knowledgeable person being labelled as an expert.

Humans are meant to wake up individually. The third dimensional dream states of protracted duality and polarity are nearly over. Let go of childlike toys, the foibles of personality, the mock dramas, the hesitant waiting for others to lead the way. The energy of the Christ consciousness is waiting to stir within each soul. The intelligence quotient demonstrating the individuality of character within each is required to open and flower.

The foundation of consciousness, which can be referenced as basic intelligence, latently suffers in humankind today from prior stress factors or fractures still being recorded in the herd-like strands of DNA interference.

Love is Energy

Lucifer speaking on Energy

Last night our brother Jésu spoke with me as I lay in a dreaming state. The meeting and the message were both vivid in their clarity. 'Everyone is provided with the abundance of life in the birthing state', he remarked. 'What are necessary steps required to strip from the essence are the layers of social imprints that retard the opportunity for people to breathe freely and see clearly. You are placed on the planet to show them what human eyes have not yet seen and their hands cannot touch.' Then he stepped away.

Love is energy. Energy is Love. The manifestations in life are many and manifold in appearance. Joy and grace are demonstrated in the experience of feeling. When humans learn to release emotions and once more embrace feelings within they will begin the process of identifying and unifying with their inner being of self we designate as soul. Today there is the given opportunity for any person to walk out of the maze of confused duality when they no longer wish to be involved with the discriminatory thinking of a wasteful modern society.

Ecstasy and agony are extreme examples of emotional areas separated within the framework of duality. What a burden was placed on the backs of humankind when the rational mind became separated from the core of internal knowing.

When the scientific gurus of knowledge declared that their patented systems of logic and reasoning were a superior arrangement to supersede the ritual and traditional procedures of religion they offered themselves as replicate new gods to replace the profligate workings of old gods.

God and gods in their entirety have never been more than imposed images instigated into the human mind. They are iconic reflections caused to catch human thought and then deified by idyllic worship. What god wherever situated can possibly assume the responsibility for introducing the breath of Love energy that sustains life in creature form? Were there any god capable to be the creative source of life then the energy of Love is no more than a manufactured product of mind demonstrating a measurable value for the sake of appearance.

As the minds of those loaded down with acquisitive egos and attached images of pretentious self-esteem tend to want to make do in human society. The idea of planetary love is a very saleable product and is eagerly sought after by those who are in some ways mentally and emotionally crippled. Is there any human situated on the planet today who can claim to be free of some supposed emotional drama inviting and exciting suppressed pain and fear?

The Love energy we speak of clothes us when we are naked of pretentious masks, bereft of any imposed addictions brought about by means of social conditioning. Consider that thinking minds are automatically neutralised whenever Love energy appears.

Love can never be wrought by thought. The energy sustaining life is beyond humanistic ideas of selfishness. To speak of giving to others unconditional love is an attempt to impose conditions onto them. The idea of unconditional love being bestowed on others collapses under the weight of its own ludicrosity, offering a stipulated ownership of variable situations. What has been compiled by errant thought processing in ego management cannot be maintained or sustained for much longer for that which is noted as given life is in a process of rearrangement.

All thought is a conditioned activity drawn from out of the reflexive cells or shallow wells of bygone memory. Therefore what people think and then say unwittingly reinforces worn out frames of prior conditioning. This only enmeshes the mind into deeper areas of denial through the overuse of compulsive repetition. It has been said of people that a lie repeated often enough will soon be taken on as a truth cemented in stone.

Is there a way out from the maze of denial that continuously breeds more lies as an excuse for personal performances that fail to measure up to expectations?

The short response is yes. This happens when people are prepared to move beyond a stalemate of crass ideas reliving past theories that are no more than a recall of old fashioned beliefs. Thus the requirement is to work our way into and through programs instilled in the brain that offer a new mind the benefit of greater understanding. What then occasions within the mind is the opportunity for appreciating silence, a measure of stillness where the clarity of future vision replaces the dysfunctional chatter so prevalent in everyday social practices.

There is a process of discovery and recovery in memory available within the psyche that requires people first to go within their selves to achieve a solemn stillness of mind. To find the divine light of remembrance we must tear away the fabric of false darkness that covers like a blanket the ignorance and arrogance of those whose overwrought minds have been ego driven to distraction.

It helps in a rearrangement of mind and memory when we can soften the illusionary fabric first with tears. Sorrow and joy are agencies developed from the same cloth. Tears can be shed for both. The internal tearing will cause the rents in the fabric of the human ego to surface and flow regardless of riven thought. Let the ego dissolve its areas of arrogance until it finds an acceptable balance within mind. Love energy waits with open arms to greet those who are able to take that first vital step of breaking through the barricade of imaged planetary pain.

Love employs greater energy offering resolvement of errant issues, which performs wonders on procedural levels well beyond human recognition of planetary values.

Love encompasses all that is incomprehensible to the human mind. The rational processing of the conscious mind is only able to grasp a proportional understanding of things that are separate from others. Wholeness in greater understanding is beyond the scope of third and fourth dimensional reasoning in mind.

Has the human mind a remembered experience of Love eternal? When Love appears to leave the planetary system, there is an accompanying heartache described as emotional pain. Where can there be any sensation of emotional pain while we are immersed in Love? Separation is a kink in the linked chain of mind that operates its quirky sequences from a localised memory bank called psyche. In the depth of the cosmic heart there can only be the realization of wholeness born from the energy of oneness.

Filling our hearts and minds with Love energy is created by emptying out all beliefs, snide influences, and diverse opinions that adversely affect the recall of innate wellbeing.

As human entities we are continually seeking yet do not find Love. Love absorbs us when we are prepared to surrender whatever is not rightly ours to possess.

Good works though praiseworthy in itself will not achieve this form of giving over, for in the manner of planetary involvement there is an ego form of management exercising choice plus the addictive ideas of freewill and choice. So learn to sit still and allow whatever is being willed onto you by the machinations of others to stultify and collapse.

Love does not ask anyone to pray. Nor does it say that we as people are expected to hold instant answers to problems that plague us. Love gives of its energy in support of life without questioning.

Love is Energy beyond Description

Love, which stands without subterfuge has no superlatives, no descriptive corollaries.

Within the arms of Love, Beauty and Truth dance in harmony. Wherever Beauty touches base, as in the heart, Truth establishes a benchmark, useful for determining future mind growth warping into rays of greater understanding.

Love constitutes being. And being offers an expression for living free. One cannot live, truly be alive, without the endorsement of Love energy.

Where is Foundation

Ensuring the cosmic mind is suitably balanced every belief is to be set aside in favour of the certainty in establishing wholeness.

Confidence or surety in mind is nurtured within the realized foundation of one self.

To locate the innate foundation signifying true self the interference of the esteemed flag of ego is to be lowered and neutralised. The nominated ego stance of superior management feeds off conditioned beliefs. So ipso facto, the less belief retained in memory the lower is the influence of ego manipulation in mind.

When you wish to benefit from a full and ripe season ahead, learn to separate the young roots of fresh growth in mind from the old muddled heap of an already vanquished society pushing for possessions.

Foundation of Consciousness

The foundation of consciousness, which can be referenced as cosmic intelligence, suffers in the minds of humankind from stress factors or fractures located in a recall of structured memory.

Every belief that has been taken on is meant to be washed away and replaced with a certainty of understanding deriving from cosmic foundation. Questions of age, questions of made over beauty, questions of perversity or suitability; all such questions are to be broken apart, realigned, and then brought together in a harmony of wholeness.

Those whose minds have gained a realization of life beyond social expectation enter into an awareness of surrounding Love energy. The purpose in living free is to establish an accord within each human system that resonates with the profoundness of eternal life.

Where is the foundation of human life?

Simply stated it is cosmic energy promoted as Love. To uncover and recover our destined glorious involvement with life and living free first we are to establish a greater understanding of that which is viable in cosmic memory. Then those who follow through behind our lead have an opportunity to endorse the production of improved health, enriched wealth in greater understanding and enduring relationships demonstrating endearing qualities.

Awakening to a New Day: Inheriting a Cosmic Mind

The foundation for a cosmic mind development activates within each person who steps up willingly to address the plate of greater understanding.

Find the glorious future held within being through releasing the old mind conditioning with its chaotic thoughts, distraught beliefs and distracted memories. Within the hidden cells or wells of the psyche that which is waiting to be revealed is a new mind and memory. A new day stands ready to inspire a fresh methodical manner of living free, an advanced way of greeting providence, with a timely preparation for engaging future eventualities.

Limiting Factors

Ignorance maintains a bench or shelf that forms blockages in inducted knowledge where a greater understanding of authenticity within the true self is hopelessly out of reach.

Arrogance in mind is fostered by circumstantial belief patterns. Beliefs in turn are fostered by the ego induced esteem system declaring for superiority over others seen as lesser than. Arrogance is brittle in structural framing and tends to break down or apart under mildly applied pressure.

Prideful people in all ignorance are condemned to fall and fail by their own displays of arrogance and superiority, which demonstrates stupidity. Such idiotic play-acting given time to fade out will invariably find its own level of despair.

Energy built from the depths of foundation does not falter when put under pressure.

Modern beliefs are a form of political kite flying, but who has control in the flight or landing? When the realization arrives that no one can ground a belief then the registered outcomes in believing remain as wild flights of fancy launched without any substance of knowing.

Beliefs are theoretical suppositions arrived at without the benefit of foundation. Collapsing belief systems create a fundamental opportunity for destructive energy within the system to surface and dissipate.

Knowledge is only proportional in any given understanding of life because its ramifications have been haphazardly built on conclusions that are without the firmness of foundation.

It is only when you are prepared to admit that worth and not value is your inner strength that you will locate your foundation. From that basic energy you can then build your future and fortune. We would call that stepping into the New Life. We would call that living free. We would call that the opportunity for humans to come to terms within their selves so that no longer do they need to argue, ridicule, or chastise others outside their being.

Love is All

Touching Life in every Aspect

That Love is All
How soft the sound
How sweet the call
Reminding us
That Love is all

Lucifer: Love energy offers certain areas of individuality. Though you cannot condense the enormity of Love you can involve yourself with certain distinctive patterns. One of those areas mentioned earlier was touch. When you put your hand out to receive Love with the willingness to touch then Love in exchange will touch you. If you refuse to put your hand out the energy of Love will not respond.

So it is probably fair to say that for human thinking Love could be seen as a responsive energy. It does not push itself onto people. So then you have to make yourself available and you are to do that without wearing defensive armour plating for mind and body protection. Love does not offer offence so has no requirement for defence.

Love is and yet is not. For to say that Love is, speaks as though something is apparent to human thought. Love is not available in that sense. Wishing or wanting things to happen now is the sign of a petulant child. Outward desire causes inward stress.

Love is not apparent to have and hold in planetary style. It is sublime. Love energy forms from the waves of the Great Ocean. Who is silly enough to say when looking at the surface or what is visible to the naked eye that what is seen is the whole of the ocean depths?

Aspects of Energy

Absorption: The energy field delivering the Great Mother Love. The energy of Love absorbs, embraces, and supports all forms of Life.

Nothingness: Can be seen symbolically as the womb of Love. Love is both giving...and forgiving.

Receptivity: Being prepared to listen for the inner call. Love energy is accessible to knowing through the vibration of inner feeling.

Dark Mother Energy: 'The male memory has had its mark made on history. The female revelation has held its stake through a reserve called mystery. Love is the embrace of All. Not contained. Not divided. Nor selective.'

Cup of Life

Blessed are those
Embracing the Rose
Whose cup of life
Is emptied of strife

Give from the heart
So tears will start
Let go of the mind
Songs of joy to find

Dreams of our youth
Start trickles of truth
To locate the lover
Learn to give over

Chapter XI.

Two Selves

On Meeting Strangers

People seek pearls and do not know how to dive
They crave diamonds and are not prepared to dig
They carry stones and cannot let go of the burden
They run around when sitting still is appropriate

Truth cannot be found for it was never lost
What do they seek, these walkers on a path
Some image, a memory, other times, other places
Empty spaces in need of constant filling
Illusion grows any flower to confuse the seekers

Meditate on the rose, the emblem of the family
Many will deny the family and in so doing
Deny the worth of self within
The family does not deny them
Only they can do that

The Mother waits with open arms
To welcome us home
Her voice is calling
Her face is in your dreams
Home is not a dream
The dream is what is presently half-lived
And taken on as real

If these words seem strange
It is because of division
A lack, a void, a need
Maintaining a dualistic separation
Between thy self, our very own stranger

Getting to Know You Series

July 2021

Finding out Who We Are

Interviewer: Where do we start?

Lucifer: There is no beginning. We are already into relationship.

Interviewer: Can we maintain pleasure within our relationship?

Lucifer: Pleasure is an attempt to block out pain by using diverse methods of mental and physical modes of escapism. It is important to understand that diversion is a tool of the superficial mind. There can be a certain amount of pleasure produced by pain in effort and conversely in the pain being constant or frequent it can be divided by measures described as pleasurable.

In extreme cases of emotional pressure, such as employing various whips of physical activity, particularly those of matters sexual, it used to be called sado-masochism. Today, we understand when it is a similar mind thing of torturous behaviour with another it has been renamed as codependency. That is something like imposing an interactive sweet poison or sour type of pain into our self and others to jointly receive a sickness benefit.

Interviewer: Can we then go beyond the cruelty of the endless cycles of emotional pushing and pulling between the sexes and even those of the same sex? Is it forever religiously ordained that male energy will maintain an aggressive stance and the female recipient when put under pressure is to be seen as a victim?

Lucifer: Women carry male energy as the male is also female orientated. With all the good intentions in the world the helpers and carers for others, intent on preserving societal standards, are condemned by their associations and their own conditioning to participate in the relevant mini-dramas through the variety of images being portrayed. Then at some stage there can be a display of role reversals so the victims of today become the aggressors of tomorrow and vice versa.

Interviewer: If people change or rearrange the images, will the recycling programs that have been performed for ages cease?

Lucifer: In any change there may be an initial suggestion of clearing or completion, but it is not necessarily so. Change like the mental divisions of pleasure may well provide a temporary relief; however, it is not a lasting release. Always in change there will be a neglect of some small area that allows a regrowth of what is being hoarded in the subconscious mental system. There may be a short period of dormancy, but after a while the cycle starts again.

An extreme example is the violence of war games followed by an aversion to troubled times where there is an arranged peaceful settlement. With war there is the manifestation of external conflict. In planetary peace, which was shattered and scattered into shards or pieces by conflict there is a steady growth working toward unity. When the pieces are not properly aligned and enjoined there is a recurrence, a triggering that comes from a malformed memory raging for revenge. Then there is a build up of subliminal tension, a subdued frustration that compulsively forms into bursts of anger, which emphatically demands attention by once more evidencing violent behaviour.

Interviewer: What is violence then?

Lucifer: Violence is the physical expression of pain that erupts from the emotional frustration of a subordinate inaction that subliminally carries a denial of self. It is caused by a glitch, a malfunction in mind processing, an inability to comprehend that which is essentially vital to achieve self-determination. These are blocks on internal issues of importance and therefore deny solutions the opportunity to give satisfactory expression to release stress driven minds. A limited aptitude to absorb pressure and encompass pain can cause a retaliatory snap, which is the sound of a breaking point.

Interviewer: Can anyone acquire the necessary information to assuage tension and encompass the limitations of the mind? Where and how should such research be carried out?

Lucifer: It has been stated that each human is unique in whatever manner of engagement is invoked. That being so then introduced material of a planetary vogue carrying a predominant influence though not accuracy, will not seat well in the reflexive portion of the psyche system that is recalled memory. The misunderstandings of life are a series of accumulated pictures or framed images stored in deep seated memory cells.

Where there is distortion, some time warping, an overlapping of parts or pieces, there is a perception, actually a misconception, which presumes there has been lack or loss. Every planetary person carries in memory frames these images of partial distortion. Humans are genetically born with them. The images are fed through the DNA and then reinforced by surrounding events, which are then absorbed like childhood memories. Most of the worrying memories from childhood are selective in presentation and inaccurate in reflection. Nevertheless, they are instrumental in causing mental conflict in adult determination.

Interviewer: We have spoken earlier of victimization in society. Would you care to give an example of how this occurs?

Lucifer: Societies carry and deliver through their differing agencies not so subtle abuse messages. There is a pecking order instigated in the varying demands of family circumstances. Reports of abuse are certainly on-carried via the media predilection with glamour afforded victim status.

These are only some parts of the formalised education systems that are bound to invoke responses from those who compulsively align themselves as victims of put upon and put down versions. By emphasising the messages of victimisation in society, the practitioners of manipulation within the wealth and health industries have created a recurrence of extreme profit margins for their own benefit.

Interviewer: How does one stop becoming a victim?

Lucifer: Start by understanding that those who label others as victims, are attempting to remove their own stigmata of pain, or wounded demeanour, by shoving the inward pressure felt elsewhere. Do not accept a parcel stamped with the label of victim. Mark the label, 'Return to sender' with a smile and hand it back unopened.

There is so much magnanimous new age talk about 'unconditional love' in the social workings of the everyday. The use of the phrase is like attempting to bluff when playing a hand of blind poker. For the proponent advocating unconditional love the fear lies…fear always lies or misrepresents…in someone calling their bluff, which means a show of cards that will disclose what it is being withheld.

80 years ago, when this presence was a small child adults recommended whistling in the dark to pretend they were not afraid. What has changed? Today the so-called leaders of beguiling instruction with their guiding hands on social wellbeing are whistling harder than ever.

Who and what are the Two Selves

Can you remember who you were before society told you what you are?

Who is aligned with the Great Mother energy.

What is a reflective process determining various levels of planetary consciousness. The hours of daily living is mainly filled with what. That leaves people little time to consider situational areas located within their being, which are not yet familiarised because the latent subconscious mind feeds from memories that have not surfaced.

Realization is an advanced tool of mental decisiveness that cannot be taught by educational methods such as curriculum teaching bounded by the falsity of suggestive reality. However, the basic fundamentals of greater understanding can be absorbed into mind and memory through a process we describe as **living free.**

Death is dissolution of what you are in flesh, not who you are in spirit. **What** is determined by planetary existence. **Who** is an inexplicable.

Being is beyond human definition: An understanding of who we are dignifies the inner essence being nominated as soul.

Who we are is the question of the moment. Each of us is more than just an enigma. The book of Life retains the record of human heritage. '**Who** we are' draws its material strength from strands and strains of DNA memory, which pertinent records are stored in hidden vaults of the human psyche.

'**What** we are' coincides more with stored memory from planetary experiences and ascribes learned knowledge as a guide to further mental advancement. What you are signifies the role the supercilious remark 'I am that I am', a pretence demonstrated in maintaining ego management. Most people in society live in a bland unsuspecting denial of who they truly are. They prefer to promote what they are or have become as reflected in the admiring eyes of others seen as less fortunate.

What you are is on display in everyday occurrences. **Who** you are is set in a deeper order of array or survey, which means your future is already planned or mapped and waiting for an ongoing delivery of events to realize an innate cognition.

Nobody needs to physically die to reach an accord within of mutual agreement. There is a recommended process achievable for survey through unifying the two selves signified as presence and essence.

Reconnection of Essence and Presence

The Angels say that the mirrors in play today are reflective of human dreaming states. In smashing the discordant mirrors of beliefs, we destruct the dreams of folly because over eons in time the intended patterns for living free have become distorted and are set in mental disarray. There is a requirement to collapse whatever is featured as an outworn past in order for a new mind of greater understanding to be assembled free of psychic entanglements hampering human growth.

The essence is like a sweet perfume that emanates from Love energy.

Two and a half million years ago as endorsed pioneers of a cosmic engagement we dropped onto the surface of planet Earth and elevated the crawling human species into walking upright by utilizing two feet. We have returned many times since then to further engage the human mind and body in advancing their limited mental programs into new levels of developed understanding.

This time we will complete a series of exercises through rearranging warped areas of biased mental framing into more balanced engagements of mind and brain devoid of plagiarized duality and polarity systems that are seriously out of whack and therefore out of contention.

Before we lift off the planet this time we will have assisted in reconnecting the human presence with its cosmic essence. Coalescence is the state of joining both presence and essence into one unified being.

The human presence precedes the awareness of essence.

Reference to Spinoza: 'The persona, which is the nominated presence, precedes the locating of essence.'

How It Will Happen

Forget the questioning how. The how will take care of its area without human interference. The cosmic pipeline to provide humans with a greater understanding of life and living free is open-ended. There is a continuous flow of energy now available that moves both ways synchronistically. Can anyone have a say on what is real in this world when every institutionalised scenario on display is a tragic mock up of affairs built on patterned beliefs?

And the ending of each deliberate act of so-called god given freewill and choice is usually a right royal fuck up! The suggested reality in mind determined by thoughts of rationality can be likened to a foggy miasma emanating from bog or swamp. Reality as such is held in locked up areas of belief called mindsets that remain sticky and gooey as caked mud.

The superpower of the United States of America operating as a headquarters for a democratic world government and spearheading a dominating global police force is close to shutting its doors. There is an energy flow now being introduced on the planet that does not allow the use of force or power to fight imaginary battles for supremacy.

Like the rumoured black holes of space the energy being promoted sucks force and power into a maw situation thus rearranging mired patterns and synergistically offering more in return. No one can maintain fire without fuel and air. So when the cosmic fire consumes the air of atmosphere to create a flare it will diminish planetary power by its own resources of greediness. Then once more lit candles of empirical power stutter to a sequential close.

We invite everyone to become mentally blindfolded and turn around. When you take the blindfold off where you are pointed is the way to locate new measures of greater understanding. The pathway is not set out deliberately for your personal use. We carry the energy to be like the wind that comes from behind and overtakes whatever is blocking the way. It can lift you up and drop you elsewhere. So use the four winds to clear your journey! Parts of you are still out in the cold and futilely putting the finger up to argue for whatever it is you know not.

Synergy is the development of coordinated energy where the product of merging allows the effective use of more energy than the combined efforts of singular ingredients. It is demonstrated by symbolizing 2+2=5. In the combined use of mental activity, it patently became known as brainstorming. However, in most cases it was a case of putting the cart before the willing horse.

With the advent of a new mind to operate freely, it first requires some small effort in brain draining accumulated rubbish. That which works in harmony with greater understanding is agreed effort. What stultifies progression in future mental movements is a locked in recalcitrant memory.

Preference for Essence

Two Genies

*As they went sojourning, a daily walk
Two genies were given to inspired talk
Agreed two heads were better than one
They then determined as a figure of fun
To put them together without much fuss
Deriving what is quoted as geni-us*

Have a preference for entering the cosmic mind into essential activity.

This discussion is about linking of the two entity/energies where the physical presence is to conform to energy we call essence, which is designated as spirit or soul. To do that the emphasis is first to be placed on the spotlighted presence, which is required to lower its exorbitant level of ego prominence. The aim is to find a mutual level of tranquillity in balance merging equally with soul.

It is not suggested the rearrangement should be seen in a form of denial of daily activity. It is marked in the form of cosmic agreement. As we have said in poetic form two heads when put together are more balanced in mutuality. Until such times as our minds are open to broaden the subject of living free our planetary situations remain suspended or static. So just like energizing a battery we need a spark of cosmic enlightenment to enter and illuminate the present day situations.

What is being asked to place on the table for consideration is a warm spark of generosity that sets the extended play into creditable action.

The glare of compromise for those who waver is similar to a deer being caught in the headlights of a car. Or like hesitating when reaching the point of no return in a given journey. Then again it can be referenced as refusing to participate in a game play of all or nothing. Perhaps it is a case of throwing caution to the wind as in for a penny in for a pound. The parting of separate ways to meld back into one principled entity/ energy is a major conundrum that defeats paradoxical thinking.

One thing is certain: having committed to diving full form into an unknown cosmic future there is no way you can go back to reclaim where you were when you first entered. Is it a form of death we offer? Only if your preference is to remain fixated on seeking out everyday mortal pleasures. The Greater Energy advise us it is a transference of mind and brain into a dimensional means of transportation, which opens the framed borders inhibiting mental progress to bring into expanded view the new cosmic horizons of the Fifth Dimension.

The day people realize they are no longer special in the planetary mind of ego is when they will discover and begin to uncover the hidden specialities the human energy carries within the outer presence presumed by scientific boffins to be effectively real.

Determining the variations between opposite and apposite: An apposite does not oppose therefore is not wilful. Duality should be seen as harmony in energy, not as contradictory in purpose, which is disposed as an opposite or opposing condition. For example, consider the dual wheels engaged on the rear axle of a truck. The paradox is that it doubles its strength in carrying a load and halves the strain or stress in lading.

A belligerent mind hears the word sound duel as combating and a mind in harmony hears dual expressed like in sharing the load.

There is one little letter of difference between opposite and apposite; duel and dual. The rational mind cannot distinguish between the differences in pronunciation that seemingly sound the same. It depends on the framed mood of the listener. If you are in an ugly mood you will hear duel and if you are in a pleasant mode you will hear dual.

Brain Drain

The mind that is overloaded or overwrought is confused and is prone to hearing insinuations of despair that are not there nor intended. So we are to clear our minds of interfering nuances. The way to do that is to practice emptying the memory in brain of belief patterns. Exercising a symbolic brain drain to remove detritus is at least the first step. That which is steeped in harmonic sequence will remain as basic fodder in contentment.

What are harmful practices from the past need to be itemized and drained forthwith. There is an old saying what is within each person is its own worst enemy. The innuendos that people are inclined to still on-carry in society are harmful to their inner system.

Inner Self Work

Lucifer Speaks

So what Lucifer would like to say is simply this: as much as we talk about the extremities of duality or the areas of polarity, we are still faced with the task of melding the necessary communication between the inner self, which is soul energy, and the planetary self, which is namely the persona dominated by ego management. So the mean point that we speak of somewhere between arrogance and ignorance is a projected requirement for a meeting between the inner self, the innate understanding of energy, and the ego self, which is being run ragged on maintaining control of planetary knowledge.

So there is a requirement for each of us to locate that middle area of balance between essence and presence. And in that mental researching we are not to give advantage to either area. What we are saying is that it is necessary to concede that ego was a required development of planetary know-how for the purpose of sustaining early survival. However, it does not carry the intuitive understanding that we are required to open and duly acknowledge resident within our inner self.

Again, it is necessary to comprehend that the external pressure or pronounced effort of the ego system is predominantly male oriented, and the internal self that offers the advisement of wisdom and beauty is female energy ordained by the Great Mother. So for us who have indicated our journey on the Rainbow Trail as a way of working back home to where we belong we are required at this time to work at marrying or merging both of these two separated areas.

To do that we have to reach an agreement that the ego presence will reduce in size from its presently projected status, and that the soul energy will assert its essence so that there is a common meeting ground and an enjoining where they unify, or as we frequently call it become as one. That is one of our principal areas of immediate work, individually and collectively. That is the pinnacle we are required to aim towards. It does not matter two hoots who you cohort with daily on the planetary scene. This work is inner self-work. You are to do it on your own. Do not expect that others will be available to carry you across the line.

Chapter XII.

Our Background & Work

We are Almost There

The sounding of sweet pipes
Will raise your head to stare
Listen and ponder
Is that a touch of Angel breath
Upon your hair
Try to recall the wonder
A memory from distant past
A summer tune or wintry blast
Invites to release all care
We are almost there

Cosmic Pioneers

Where we as cosmic pioneers are situated at present and where we descended from.

Luxor represents the Torchbearer. The role of torchbearer pioneers the lighted way in developing human benefit in achieving greater understanding.

Luxor, an adapted pen name for a beyond cosmic entity/energy, the Unnamed One, habituating Earth as a human presence, is a version of the more formal title, Lucifer. Its Latin meaning denotes the bearer of the light of Intelligence. He carries aloft the ignited torch of blue flame. Consider that there are many others on the planet working in conjunction so we do not proceed alone.

All religions can be seen as breakaway satellites formed from the orbit of the central sun. All are presently staged as stalled plateaus and cyclical in movement. They each contain only partial elements of Truth. The torchbearer comes to Earth periodically to light the way to progress greater understanding.

Luxor: This present day journeying or solitary type sojourning, whichever description you prefer, has been ongoing for the past 25 years with my working partner, Jézel. We have been dedicated in working on suitable methods to bring human consciousness to new levels of greater understanding; to awaken and align the rational mind of humans with what is to be the next shift or lift of conscious energy. We are presently based and operate globally through utilizing an Internet connection situated on the Gold Coast, Queensland, Australia.

Why are we stationed here and what is our intentional purpose in broadcasting cosmic material globally? Humans en masse are programmed to enter a new level of intelligent existence, to be re-positioned cosmically, which particular area has been nominated as the Fifth Dimension.

The studious work of developing cosmic understanding has absorbed us day by day, week by week. Even so, year by year to put together in print a resume of entity/energy levels that exist not only in the cosmic field, but also in extended fields and even beyond fields where there are greater beyond fields still to come into cosmic play.

Jézel is a pen name indicating the connective entity of Jésu with the compelling energy of Love.

Jézel: Initially our operative skills in cosmic connections began when Luxor started to receive distinctive messages in his head from unknown quarters back in 1993. He was then in his 57th year. His planetary background was mainly involved in mercenary activities, which did not prepare him for the dimensional worlds of the cosmos his mind and brain was about to encounter.

These new forms of communicative voices advise him on future and past happenings of planetary development and rearrangements that contradicts much of what science sets down as evolutionary procedures.

He began engaging in brief encounters with interesting people, who on the surface were ordinary looking but sub-culturally their lives were very different from the usual run of the mill society. He was required to share time with them and exchange small understandings of hidden worlds, operating beneath the thinly veiled fabric of modern civilization.

Then all of a sudden through heat emanating from his hands he became a conveyor of healing energy without requiring touch. He could act as a clearing agent for some people with serious ailments through removing mental pain that was lodged in their deep-seated memory banks. He gradually became aware that it was cosmic Angels whose voices he had nominated as 'they' were using him to do this specialized type of work.

During this time, Luxor was compelled to research many library shelves and New Age bookshops to gain esoteric understandings of the background to religions, metaphysics, philosophy, and sciences involving parapsychology, anthropology, and such related matters. All of these carried areas of information that had never previously interested him.

Much that he was led to read was interesting though much he discounted as outmoded or was moved to reinterpret because his mystery teachers, whom he instinctively felt were benign, would use the material to show an outline of a larger picture; demonstrating how human focus, being of narrow bent at best, tended to grasp onto immediate issues and therefore denies association with more advanced material that is meant to be opened and used for greater purpose.

Breaking through Barriers

In mental experimentation with the psyche Luxor was led further into visionary experiences, past and present, which would provide an expansion of mind that gained even greater purpose in understanding.

He was shown in a series of graphic visions the workings or machinations of diverse strata building, planetary, universal, and cosmic. It was work performed by Angels and other cosmic beings of varying strains, which included Ancients, a male energy force who were responsible for the building of universal planets. They were the initial creators and promoters of the specified creature form called Man, plus organizing the stocking of flora and fauna on this planet with the aid of elemental creatures.

D'Taan continues the Recount

Then in 1995, Luxor reconnected with a previous acquaintance, Jézel, who is mutually associated in this work area where they became intent on finding the location of inner selves. They first met in a little theatre play house in a small country town of Caboolture in 1988. Their newly advanced friendship in 1995 was built on an agreed understanding they were to use the mind of each other as sounding boards to delve into respective psyches and examine, by bringing into light, that which was subliminally being withheld from rational vision and explanation.

Luxor again takes over the Recounting of our Historic Journey

Amongst many memories of past performances, including times spent in Lemuria, Atlantis, and even further back when star ships roamed the galaxies, what we discovered and uncovered were advanced material programs ready to be shared with other beings of like interest on planet Earth today.

What was introduced for our understanding is that there are some 500,000 such designated characters situated on the planet available for interactive service with others of similar cosmic background. At this stage most are still sleepers, but some are already awakening and working studiously for the benefit of humane causes. We would consider very few are fully aware of who they really are at this time or what deeper understandings though still dormant lie in wait to guide their futuristic work.

A major event for us occurred on 10/11/96 where we participated in a small group meditation celebrating the 11 11 momentum. We experienced a vital re-connection, a communicative awakening to greet our immediate Divine family, and realise our far-reaching purpose in being once more placed on the planet. After the awakening of who we are to cosmically represent in human form we were shut down temporarily for just short of a year.

Then in late 1997, the voices in our heads made themselves identifiable as Angels and they referred to Lucifer as a friend. Much of our training since then has been delivered by Angel discussions. Though neither Jézel nor I, both endowed with beyond cosmic strains of energy, have come from Angel stock.

In October 1997, another major breakthrough occurred when Jézel suddenly became an open channel for an assortment of cosmic beings, which included Angels, star beings, some of the cosmic builders we call Ancients, and Elemental stock, Fairies, Elves, and other little people.

For many years we probably averaged twice a week hourly discussions with a vast range of entity/energies, including Mother, Father, Sister, Brother Lines of energy, each area coming from varying strains, with stories of their involved roles in the functioning of planet Earth and their ongoing input into furthering human development. Presently for the most part, we utilize our internal messaging for further elucidation.

We have tabulated these cosmic greetings and discussion type meetings with many entity/energies on a series of tape recordings and for a short time on video tape recordings. As we came to realize the material being offered was for future book purposes we began transcribing and collating whatever material we considered relevant for further research.

We now have a huge library of recorded information, much more than thousands of hours pertaining to past happenings on this planet and in the cosmos, over-viewing events of interest happening today, with outlines of further proceedings destined to occur in the near planetary future.

This information when broadcast globally will spin the keepers of planetary knowledge to land on their unbalanced heads. Planetary knowledge in the near future will have few basic footholds left to clamber up what has always been a tenuous cliff face of planetary beliefs and ideals.

We, this small core of pioneers installed on planet Earth, have broken through the veil that has hidden and forbidden Love. As such we are bonded in Love with the Great Mother energy. We have been given the keys to understand the three principles therefore we are set the task of relaying to human suffrage the cosmic understandings maintained in **Truth**, **Equality**, and **Unity**. By such means as Internet exchanges and written material people will gradually come to terms with understanding who they are and the greater purpose in which they are bonded.

Breaking through Outmoded Barriers

It was in the hidden areas of the psyche, labelled occult, where we first directed our prescient intention to break through the masks and uncover whatever mysteries were hindering the mental growth of planetary people. We were intent on developing a precise mind cleansing process, thus ignoring the efforts of transcendental meditation, or NLP type self help courses advocating power of the mind as a be all, end all. We opted for seeking a purposeful exploration of the psyche memories resident behind the mirrored ego mind maintaining beliefs.

We knew instinctively there was more to uncover about the history of the human species than religion or science proclaimed. Thus we refused to settle for less than what we considered to be a bigger picture of life.

Eventually through using a series of devised visual techniques we broke the seals containing the conscious human memory to locate further information beyond what are termed subconscious/unconscious mind levels and stepped willingly into pioneering roles intent on exploring the vast void of cosmic nothingness.

What we discovered were greater programs for human endeavour waiting to be uncovered, ratified, and delivered to the minds of those seeking fulfilment through a comprehensive survey of that which is unknown. We then built a small foundation of realization within ourselves from the advanced understandings placed on offer. We shared these qualities of genuine style living with others who were also in some way pioneering, ready and willing to move into revealing the next levels intended for communal involvement.

A greater understanding of Life and living free in the ever present will soon leave archaic religions and scientific speculation behind, as they are merely shaky mental platforms seeking credibility in this linear age denoting space and time. As this planet and its accompanying creatures move into their next level of cosmic dimension, a programmed eventuality anticipated to occur in the next few years, a new mind built on the certainty of a cosmic foundation in life becomes available for access.

That which is fated or destined for humankind, in a relayed series of sequential posts or positions, will surely and securely anchor the present day mind suffering from the contamination of an overactive ego, back into unified levels of a more expansive intelligence.

Contrary to popular beliefs held fast in ego manipulation the everyday mind does not have need of defensive barriers called protection. It is enough to say the domineering ego has a tendency to compulsively overreact, overreach, and thus lose its capability for stability when placed under pressure. When it is cosmically dragged back to relocate into suitable formations of balance a greater realisation of Love and Intelligence becomes firmly established within all future cultural happenings. Meanwhile destiny is playing out the closure of this third dimensional planetary phase, where subjective forms of mental slavery are deliberately affecting the future growth of human minds and memory.

Background Sketch of Discovery

A background sketch in accessing a New Mind that leads to the discovery and future recovery of the cosmic heritage, which was initially designed for the building of the human species.

Let us say from the outset that the few in numbers who played the role of self-realizing guinea pigs in these pioneering exercises did not use mind-bending drugs of any kind. Small amounts of white and red wine were consumed for the purpose of relaxing the rational mind, which was subject to rash moments of anxiety when their ego systems became aware we were intent on trekking outside or beyond the standard limitations of mental comfort zones.

We were cognisant with the fact that many experimenters had used different drugs over the years to alter mental states of what is nominally called consciousness. Drug usage of any kind cannot provide the clarity of mind necessary for deep-seated memory explorations of the psyche. Like generalized reporting that comes from the hearsay of disturbed or distorted memory of events drug assistance only gives a simulated version of actuality, an appearance of form for what is termed in practised science as reality.

Through using particular processes of selective remembering, something like a H. G. Wells mental time tracking machine sent into a DNA tunnel, we explored different methods of purposefully accessing the human psyche. In our meditative travels, we met on several occasions dead end walls in blocked alleyways and retraced our steps partially to attempt breaking through using a variety of methods to regain access. Perseverance in effort eventually broke down the mental barriers of resistance and we achieved the breakthroughs to uncover what are forgotten memories beguiling humankind.

The memory cells in psyche we succeeded in opening contained vital material pertinent to a forgotten past, which being unavailable for modern distribution denies present day mind advancements into greater levels of intelligence. The time is ripe for humans to upgrade the limitations of standards imposed by the institutionalised minions of societies, whose everyday platforms built from religious beliefs are decaying fast because they have reached their use by date.

Here is an opportunity being given openly to move interested people intellectually beyond the trite conditioning that we call moral education. Scientific knowledge carries a series of faults that impede and block new levels of greater understanding, and in so doing peremptory retard the mental progress of developing children.

These records from the past may sound like souped up hieroglyphics found by some raiders of a lost ark, but we assure you neither religion nor the dramatis personae of scientific guess workers can play a leading role in what we relate for the benefit of communal advancement.

When the specialized cosmic information we received was inserted into rationalized thinking and merged with the present day levels of reticent knowledge our minds exploded like starbursts, a nova rosa in colour and sound. When the cosmic dust settled what was embedded in mind and memory were greater programs of living Intelligence, which had upgraded our mental faculties into more advanced levels beyond thought we nominate as greater understanding.

We are able to present a comprehensive program, an understanding of human heritage and purpose in life that will confound present day experts and encapsulate ordinary minds into raptures of childlike awe and wonderment as their true heritage of spiritual development is revealed.

Experimental work in the Psyche

In the infancy of developing new levels of mental growth into a greater understanding of energy flow we initially engaged with the rational mind of ego sense to question the validity of its operational belief patterns. For our part it was largely experimental work because we discarded any recorded suppositions of popular frameworks of belief that might be used for the purpose of unverifiable argument. In effect we disregarded already developed new age mindsets held in our small discussion group as not being worthy of substantiation without first being subjected to a much closer critical examination.

Like miners digging for hidden gold we were intent on locating passages or veins of fresh information that would allow us the means to develop a deeper exploration of mind and an unexplored understanding of the human psyche. We figured the psyche was like an abandoned **mind** field of memories forsaken recently by medical science when drug profiteering overcame any sincere research into advancing more serious philosophic measurements of brain development.

We became very successful in cleaning and clearing out of our mental systems stressed areas of non-productive material held in abeyance in the subconscious strata of memory. While we continued to probe for errant beliefs caught fast in dualistic programming, mutated messages from no fixed address in memory continued to bubble up onto a surface level. This enabled us to eliminate waste products of unratified belief, which had previously been trapped in the subliminal memory lines, referenced scientifically today as DNA strands and strains.

On this basis we operated the practice of mental self-clearing for a period of five years. Through using volunteers and ourselves seeking more developed understanding we continued to sluice the overriding muck held in human memory by out of date belief patterning. Through maintaining a dogged perseverance that was continuously subjected to a variety of emotional challenges we eventually struck gold.

Instead of only clearing out our mental systems of rubbish material, we discovered that given a free flowing opportunity pendulums do indeed swing from whatever volition compels them. Suddenly there was a reverse influx occurring where we began to receive mental correspondence containing information that was not connected or reliant on planetary knowledge. Somehow we had become linked into an exchange system that we describe as envelopes or pleats issuing from those of greater understanding resident in the vastness of the cosmos.

One of the many advices for future human resolution was shown to us in an acquired art form portraying harmlessness as a future requirement for demonstrating the benefits that can be derived from mental balancing.

Errant Patterns of Planetary Training

As the ongoing recorded material is translated and produced it will be instrumental in rearranging the fashionable but errant patterns expounded in planetary knowledge. What is being maintained in modern religious and scientifically trained diatribe dispensed by institutionalised authorities is destined to crumble and break asunder.

The biased cant of religion and the unstructured bridges of misconstrued knowledge framed in scientific conjecture are to be burned into ash through the cleansing flames of greater intelligence. The strictured mind gaps contained in credulous belief patterns maintaining the suppurating wounds of mental pain and fear are being repealed. These patented areas of past indulgences will first be opened and then cleansed and closed with a healing balm, the Energy of Love, derived through the application of cosmic resourcefulness.

The rational or conceptual mind was programmed to initially work from imparted information obtained through the intake of senses. This method of absorption and following observation in its primary phase was instinctively used for human survival. The building of protective methods to maintain survival formed from mental imagery where developed reason was confronted with mutual concerns. Banded efforts of group mentality were stronger and more effective than pursuing individual efforts. In this manner societies were introduced by the clustering of small groups with a common distribution of provisions amongst tribal people.

In time the leaderless groups, because of infighting, recognised that their form of existence was becoming chaotic and debilitated the energy of the tribe. So they as a group gave power to the strongest and charged them with protecting the weak, which in those times were the pregnant and nursing mothers and small children. In this way progressive power systems were built into the memory banks of people and so evolutionary type processing of modern societies had its beginning.

So the flamboyant stories of anthro-apologetic flavour, such as various branches of science, would have credulous people believe what was conveyed without questioning. What is not obvious to science, the collective think tanks of practised measurement in all things physical, is that memory for survival and of survival were programmed into the human system well before humans began to experience conditioned life as it appears to the limited five senses. How else would the initial species, malformed in various body parts as they arrived into the third dimension, have survived?

It is obvious that newborn babies instinctively breathe, cry, and suck for sustenance without any prior training. Surely the instinctive methods of birth arrival are programmed because there is an electromagnetic type of shock induced into creature birthing that is not of material substance. Then there is a survival response of what is deemed to be natural causes.

The varying portions of childhood expression can be advanced by supporting systems, but whether the initial aid is a future help or hindrance is not open to question in medical systems, which invariably erase or gloss over wanton mistakes we are cosmically advised is human error that lacks in understanding.

Chapter XIII.

Lucifer Essays

There is No God

*There is no god
What's that you say
Is that to mean
I keep my knees clean
And no longer pray*

*There is no god
What a blessed relief
Here's to the day
When people can say
Release that silly belief*

*There is no god
No sanctified Geist
So reduce the cost
By giving each priest
The nod to get lost*

There is no god
Scatter the chaff
Tell the people, hey
There is a New Day
Join in a merry laugh

There is no god
Well that's a relief
Let's relay Truth
And decry belief

There is no god
Where is the proof
Neath scamming faith
There is the living truth

FOR THERE IS NO GOD

The Call Within

If you are receiving the call within to be a player in advancing world circumstances then through the developing of a greater understanding within, you can assist in straightening out diffident matters plaguing human delivery in the everyday. Then let us join together to work at tidying up those stray loose ends. It is time for lost children to realize their worth, emanating from a long lost heritage.

We are to come to the Great Mother with an empty plate and eat what is put on or provided for sampling before we ask for more. So do not get ahead of thy Self. Make sure our Self is prepared for the 'call within'. Until we hear that call loud and clear, continue to make our **selves** ready.

Let us backtrack a little bit in time and talk about knowledge as a mind development program for human conditioning, which preceded the availability of greater understanding we are drawing upon from Cosmic Intelligence today. Between the two planes or levels there is a gap that has to be filled with a linking of realization, otherwise there cannot be a smooth transition made into the more expansive measures of processing and progressing the Product.

There are three areas, recognition, realization, and greater understanding we are to become au fait with to become true representatives of the Great Mother on planet Earth. So let us start with our childhood where we learnt the ABC of forming words, then moved on to encounter simple arithmetic and then learning periods of more involved grammar and mathematics.

Following that, there were logistics and more advanced forms of grammatical expression until some of us eventually completed our studies in the senior year. Then some moved to engage tertiary levels. The first time a lecturer gets up to introduce a new subject on a tertiary level and someone remarks that it does not agree with what they learnt in senior grade the lecturer will probably tell them that senior grade only prepares them for further education. It does not give them a broader understanding of future work programs.

The realization that you are required to embrace to reach your next level of cosmic understanding is that trained knowledge belongs with planetary thinking. It has no difference or more elevated significance in its patterned frames than what you received in early training, because whatever is of worldly produce has a final or completion stage. In other words knowledge assists in daily livelihood, but it is limited in taking you further when it comes to breaking through the mundane rituals of belief and its accompanying mindsets that lock down mental advancement. Because these patterns are subject to polarity and its subordinate duality in choice its results lack substance in forming balanced measures. It can assist you though in moving forward in daily life, but towards what ends?

In all of these argy-bargy syndromes of patterned living, there is the dominant ego involvement that pushes people this way and that into differing areas of competition that are without balance. When your study days of learning are completed and you go into the work force you will be told to forget what tertiary education had to say because the real world is about adapting to work skills, which is akin to engaging in survival tactics. So the wheel has turned a full circle, because was it not survival that you were about from the very first day you drew breath?

The realization that planetary knowledge has a cut off point where no learned or erudite person, regardless of their background of training skills, can proceed beyond, is tantamount to us being willing and able to take that further step into greater understanding. It is necessary to concede a number of these points we offer for discussion if you wish to progress your mental faculties into working through interrelated cosmic zones.

So when you have the realization that there is a cut off point then to move beyond that you have to leave off or let go the childhood mentality demonstrated by humans of all ages. Then you are ready for a further step to be taken. Leaving behind what is no longer suitable for purposeful use moves you into a work field that we call greater understanding. It is an area for study that is far deeper than programmed belief systems and certainly beyond the human recall limited to rationalised memory.

Intelligence comes from greater energy that covers all aspects of planetary and cosmic durability. To link into Intelligence requires a lessening of the grasp for further knowledge in the interest of promoting do-ability. To further your knowledge in empirical matters has no vested meaning or future interest unless it is coupled with the energy that provided human intelligence.

When you are able to say, 'I leave my childhood playthings behind me without regret and I stand ready to enter into a state of adulthood as a prelude to us establishing Divine Womanhood', then the greater energy will link through mind to make its connection.

The future work that we are required to do can only be set into requisite patterns through us releasing old patterns of childhood pique that no longer carry value. It does not mean you have not gained benefit from those learning experiences. What is suggested, with these new areas humans are entering into, is that those old patterns left remaining act as blocking agents in memory; for them to be still regarded as standard fare will not fit the cosmic bill.

To move beyond the influence of ego patterning there has to be a cut off point. We have called that shift in consciousness realization, which can also be referenced to the Call Within; likening the situation of leaving one shore behind and journeying a short distance to arrive at a more advanced destination.

So when we willingly accept the realization that the life we have led until now is a closing chapter then we will be ready to begin our newly allotted program to access the Product. The knowledge we carry is beneficial for now because it gives us a certain amount of street smarts, but the information we are to receive will have nothing whatsoever to do with mental cunning or superiority, which are two of the major linchpins engaged in supporting ego society.

If You have a Light, Shine It

In regards to the greatest minds operative in this world of societies today, until such times as they are able to move beyond areas of localised rationality, they are no more capable of being able to understand what is the causation of disturbances occurring on the planet today than any small child. A child has as much understanding of what is presently happening globally as the greatest of brains trained in studying the material world.

Simply put, that which is occurring circumstantially is beyond any human mental levels of observation. So to come to terms with the planetary shift it is necessary to drain your mind of faulty knowledge to be able to accept what is happening around you in the everyday. What if this rational world built of ideas and beliefs were to suddenly explode and vaporise? What would matter to you?

We are asking what would happen if you became an ambassador for the Divine Mother and said to somebody, 'I am going to tell you something unheard of that will blow open your mental horizons'. So you tell them about friends you met being able to converse with the Divine family and Angelic levels in the cosmos, plus acknowledging Ancient energy who were creators of this planetary system.

People will go to a Star Wars movie and they will collectively pay heaps of money to be shown a mock up of a sometime bedtime story about cosmic aliens. Yet they are each carrying portions of the greatest life story in living memory unconsciously within their being at this moment.

They keep it locked up and guarded tightly behind dummy spits of ego arrogance and ignorance. In this sense Jesus spoke about the Pharisees being dogs in the manger. He basically said, 'When they cannot hear what you are to offer they won't let anybody else hear you either'. So if you have a light burning bright within, be prepared to shine it regardless of wayward interference.

Iconic Gods with Clay Feet

Those who rejected Love and instead chose hate
For them Lucifer will happily clear their slate
How stupidly dumb are those of scientific bent
Who ridiculously lay claim to being intelligent

We have no interest in aligning with any so-called creator type beings masquerading as the source of life. Religions with their rigmaroles of pomp and traditional ceremonies and rituals are collapsing and thus departing from the human banks of memory. In their stead will arise a new level of social consciousness dedicated to the three principles of **Truth, Equality**, and **Unity**. These principles and understandings are part and parcel in the minds of the new children being born on the planet. In some previous words attributed to Jesus two thousand years ago, 'A little child will lead them'.

Entity/Energies of Interference

So let us talk for the moment about other entity/energies, those who have had their day, their say, and have gone repentant or otherwise on their less than merry ways. What we are given to know of their exploits in the manipulation of earthly matters is only a portion of a much larger picture. Yet what little understanding we are required to impart of the overall picture concerning human development will devastate the errant religious orders that still exist on this planet today.

Christianity has been built on the premise that as Jesus was considered by some to be the Messiah who arrived and was not recognised as such then the recordings of the Old Testament with its early stories told by Semitic prophets must in some way be seen to be valid. In the supplementary New Testament Jesus is portrayed as the only son of god and a saviour come to Earth to comfort and welcome home to heaven those prepared to believe in him.

Let us say clearly to all those with ears that wish to hear. There is no supreme god, no heaven, or here after, except as an illusionary dream for those who want to believe in worship and prayer having value, and those who have vested interests in having others believe in those errant values. It is ridiculous to suggest that ineffable energy as Jésu carries, being presented in planetary style as the entity Yeshua, would see some value in claiming the immortality image of a god when eternal energy flowed freely through his very veins.

Gods with Feet of Clay

Each and every god worshipped by humans on planet Earth has demonstrated feet made of clay. That means they carry an iconic image and as such are caught up as earth bound entities who just like humans must wait for the day of their reckoning and their release from the state of dominion. Down through the ages those deemed as gods were projections emanating from greater entity/energies. They were visitors who lost their main connection and thus were denied contact with their initial programs and programmers.

So they are not gods of creation or even ascended masters as their devotees would have people believe. They are poor imitations of what they pretend to represent as all reflections that warp out of distinction must be. Yes, they have carried some energy in the past. It would have been a lot less without foolish people giving away a share of their energy fields to an imaged reflection they saw as being superior to themselves.

However, it gives worshippers of certain faiths the opportunity to spurn and put blame onto others whom they consider are less fortunately placed than their particular selves. These maladjusted people can be easily recognised in society because they carry aloft the foolish banners of suspect humility and compassion regarding others they see as less fortunate. So when these arrogant type people, smug in their religiosity or secularity, reach the top of the pyramid in a superior fashion, small though the elevation may be, they are obligated to invent a perspective of god sense for their continued benefit in controlling the lives of others.

Beliefs

Do people ever consider, let alone suspect, what locks their earthly frame onto this particular planet? What causes the cycles of death and rebirth that condemns each person to maintain their shoulder to the grinding wheel of subjective living on the planet Earth? People have been trained into obeying without consideration different forms of belief! Whether that early training is cemented into either believing one or disbelieving another it makes no difference. The duality of the rational mind works both ways and initially every child in being born immature cannot resist their fragile minds being trained to think in terms of opposites.

People have been suckered into believing in opposing ideas of right and wrong, good and bad, true and false, male and female in mind and body sense, the list would appear to be endless, but there is an end approaching to settle such foolish arguments that continually cause havoc in disagreements.

Beliefs are no more than mock-up images, devised methods of temporary planning, implemented by minds intent on confusing others for the sake of singular profit taking. When these so-called half truths, so subtly endorsed by the esteemed patterns of egomania, are solidly implanted amongst other variable images of the mental systems that are locked down mindsets, where the likes of wild horses cannot pull them apart.

Human Heritage

The following material is a circulated article addressed to people on planet Earth by those who are engaged in developing greater levels of understanding by utilizing cosmic standards of conjecture and contemplation.

Understanding the heritage of the human species is paramount in appreciating fresh happenings applicable to accepting a role in future cosmic consciousness.

Cosmic consciousness: the unexplored depth of hidden waters discerning human progress. It contains vital material supporting future mind development.

The greater energy humans carry within their latent brain systems cannot die and with the awakening of the human mind to its true heritage and purpose then planetary frames of religious persuasion and scientific hubris cannot survive as pitiful lies for much longer. The torch that Lucifer brings carries the Blue Flame bearing new levels of greater understanding to those prepared to listen. The new wave of energy arriving on the planet will burn the dross of perceived duality out of the human mental system.

That which people call the now should be referenced as the functional. It is a filmed layer of tissue that covers a greater expanse of knowing relating to cosmic memory. The so-called enlightened personnel of esteemed varieties, whether they are seen as scientific, religious, or educational are on loan to satisfy the whims of superior people. Those who invariably carry compassion (pity) for others seen as being less fortunate only massages opportunities to maintain their own glorified comfort zones.

Their self-assumed roles of leadership plunder those less fortunate into worshipping a monotheistic symbolism of god for those religiously bent, or to the scientific pretension of another god sense called evolution, which they say works wonders to benefit the development of humankind.

In these imaginative ways they maintain an advantage over those who have been trained since childhood into states of unquestioning subordination that knows no different.

We do not offer enlightenment to those people intent on finding spiritual answers. In many ways their tasking efforts to find whatever goal they are seeking is the journey of the fool. What we offer is an understanding of nothingness to clear the rancid atmosphere pervading human consciousness. Intelligence promotes an immersion movement beyond the dearth or darkness of planetary ignorance to develop a greater understanding of emerging cosmic life. More accurately it is like a brain drain clearing of the rational mind of beliefs, a cleaning out of vain ego strictures, which in the main have done no more than present a serial display of dramatised mini-deaths.

These deaths of ego frailty are to be replaced with fresh forms of cosmic memory release. No one will mourn the passing of ignorance presently occupying space in the human brain. Ignorance does not offer oblivion from pain though it is oblivious to circumstances that cause strife in daily life. If strife can be named in a planetary sense then it is something that has outlived its area of usefulness and will perish of its own accord through a marked lack of attention to detail.

We offer nothingness as a remedy to release the ills and chills of burdened society. No **thing.** And in various stages of acceptance the minds of people shall be cleared and live freely of harmful disturbances. The human brain already carries the potential of a greater energy awaiting its moment of arrival to succour an enduring human relationship of endearing quality. To use a cosmic term the dormancy seated inside each person, that which is not yet awakened, is Love energy. Do not seek for rationality or logic in the material we are required to relay.

An awareness of the torch that carries the Blue Flame will awaken the light of the ecstatic fire within each system. It is energy offering realisation within the accepting mind that forms from an array of cosmic levels of Intelligence. There is nothing to do except open your arms and release your mind. There is nothing physical you or anyone can do to enhance mental understanding. Sit still and allow the undoing of mental knots in mind, denials that are no more than encrusted beliefs, a hangover from distant memories that were false in the telling and cannot find any sense of value by wasted means of retelling.

While you run away the awakening energy of Love on offer will not chase. Where you choose to run and hide there is no concern. Can anyone escape their true self by a continuation of rutted denial? Can human destiny ordained in the cosmic annals be denied or refuted by vain ego?

Many humans live in the mental state of a feral animal. Their senses are heightened, magnified by the fear of imaginary pain. What began as a concentrated effort towards reaching states of perfection has become paranoia by a pinpointing stab into the unfocused mind. Be assured, it is okay for the continued pressure will relent when a new mind is deemed acceptable.

For many on the planet the grip of fear is necessary as a prelude to their awakening. Throw out protective vanities. Stand mentally naked within the light of your being. Let go of the outworn tools of your religious and quasi-scientific teachings. All they ever did was provision a protective covering to benefit a few to the detriment and harmful imagery of many.

Professed reality as expressed and endorsed scientifically is situational. Therefore, it can be moved into further awareness or replaced as circumstances dictate. If neither shift is suitable then the mind can wander elsewhere and the perceived situations may then alter to suit other occasions.

What is being offered to gullible truth seekers in society as veritable beliefs, works to ensure that science is seen as credible in any number of whoopee-do-lies to please the vanity of their captive audiences. These are their stories that enable authorised wheeler-dealers to cheat admiring supplicants of advanced measures of health and wealth.

Stepping back to see a bigger picture will allow the themes of reality to be seen as no more than a series of hand-me-down mindsets from other times, which continue to capture the minds of people in framed cages of ignorant acceptance.

When there are no longer superiority/inferiority factions of duality to plague sensibility then there is no further separation; thus the end to internal suffering occurs as an understanding of wholeness arrives.

We say it is time to seek within stored memory to identify personally with whom humans as a species are meant to be. Then the wholeness within will be distinct from the collateral damage constantly fed to people by the dissembling media sources, which periodically overload the strained senses of their readers with errant rubbish.

A Need In Deed to Know

Softly you come, with a need
To know of thy hidden part
Slightly wanton in the greed
To feel the rush of water start

Are we to press the promised key
Would turn the chains and locks
Grant each mirrored wish to see
Inside the closed Pandora's Box

Within thy self are truths to know
The die is long since cast and set
How sweet the taste of inner glow
How wide the sweep of cosmic net

Chapter XIV.

Epilogue

When our tasks on the planet are completed, when and where we eventually return to Home, once more to come awake and rise to greet with our Divine Families, to hear the accolades and applause offered to us from our extended relationships with Angels, will we not look back on these squalid type planetary adventures as some form of a dreaming state?

Or will that which we have achieved be acknowledged in the cosmos, at least to those who willed us to venture, as a vital contribution in the determined march towards achieving the ongoing goals of living spirit, an ultimate striving for wholeness/goodness, which we can only acknowledge and endorse as a consummation of Love Energy?

One more piece of embroidered fabric is truly woven into the tapestry of an eternal design referenced as the Greater Plan, with the express purpose of rearranging and upgrading existing cosmic programs.

One more explanatory chord resounds in the composing of a divine orchestration, a celestial symphony, which in the musical accord of the spheres demonstrates a greater and clearer picture of a colourful destiny; one that is filled with a rhapsody of sound interspersed with the depths of silence emanating from the Great Ocean.

Summary

Learn to turn your head and look behind you. A new day, nominated as the fifth dimension, promising a new life in living free is rising to demonstrate its splendour.

The **Product** we speak of and distribute for greater understanding involves advancement as an uplifting of human consciousness, an upgrading of human contribution that involves the use of Intelligence on a grander scale than the outworn precincts of stale knowledge. Here is an opportune moment to enter a period of what is termed a quickening of time as part in an ongoing global plan we anticipate will be concluded in less than ten years.

What and **who** is to be presented first as a beautiful story of Love and Intelligence prevailing in a rearrangement of cosmic patterning, which will be acted out planetary-wise for people of all nations as a closing chapter to the outdated third dimension. Be among the first to welcome in the arrival of a series of fresh beginnings in communal sharing and caring called the New Day.

Unifying with the Greater Energy

We are aware as it has been revealed to us that the Greater energy, though they call the shots for the cosmic rearrangement of Earth and its peopled creatures, cannot fire the enthusiasm of most laissez faire type humans. That deed has to be seen to be done on a planetary level. To inspire enthusiasm, to demonstrate personal willingness, people are to realise that the rewards of living free of impositions are inside each and every one of us. Until people can grasp there is a level of greater understanding available they are condemned to continue living the sour dregs of a distilled planetary dream.

When you feel within your **self** the call to become a player in advancing world circumstances beyond the pain and fear that is prevalent today; through personally developing a greater understanding of who you are as an initial step, then you can ably assist in straightening out a variety of diffident matters in society that still plagiarise and beggar the somnolent human mind.

What can you do to assist in Human Development?

First of all do not doubt the quality of energy you carry within your very being. The emphasis on living free should be placed on nobody in particular! We are all equal. Our work is set in realizing there is a vibration of harmony in togetherness. As there are no beginnings we are already set into play. Before we can assist others we first are to bring ourselves into the accord of oneness. The melody of living free is within.

Speaking with a representative of Greater Energy recently he stated that no one on the planet qualifies for a plus or what is called a tick of approval. So it is an open field of ripened lushness in mind and memory just waiting for the cosmic crop to be harvested to benefit humanity as a whole. Where are the projected cosmic workers on the planet willing to apply their shoulder to the wheel of human discovery and recovery?

Wondrous Events

Wondrous events placed on call
Past and present, future, all
Unfolding now before our eyes
What we are able to surmise
Is not false treaty nor reality
That which is on show is destiny

Chapter XV.

Preview of 'The Star Within'

The Future of Womanhood

Now is the time indentifying and realizing. The Divine Mother energy as we are ready to introduce her beauty and wisdom to the people of the planet.

The basic cause that we are *involved* with is providing people with a greater understanding of living free, promoting the female energy of the Great Mother, and the emanating strength in embracing Love energy. As such we are here to further the cause of female advancement through diving into our designated areas of planetary work.

Our dialogue as always demonstrates the strength there is available in mental growth and human development offering communal benefits. Our involvement does not include getting caught up in the dragnet of wasted planetary beliefs. Thus the children of the Great Mother are on the move to clarify the bullshit retained in shibboleths. Do not bother to enquire who the children are by naming, for we are they who acknowledge our dedication to Love energy.

The episodic goddess period of glamour and grandeur has failed to evince sufficient worthiness in mind and memory to continue. So its entity/energy range of activities is to retire from any further interference with the playing fields of future female advancement.

All of those hate-filled lies of religious and scientific persuasion, using implausible stories to explain their versions of creative life, were manufactured to bolster the role-playing of dire male superiority. The lies have consistently been embellished upon and used to contain and undermine the correct roles assigned for female participation. The new faces that are due to appear on the global stage are designated to play out in a communal sense the beneficial production we nominate and declare as DIVINE WOMANHOOD.

The lies that were spread by authoritarian misogynists were always reprehensible and are no longer deemed applicable.

Women are to take their appropriate places in society and communal affairs with the quiet dignity that their long held back contributions to civil practices deserve.

What is required in societies today for the broader benefit of functional development in communities are any number of female voices promoting a more comprehensive understanding of the complex energy located in womanhood. Seemingly uncoordinated, even unrecognisable and subject to denial at this time, there is a groundswell of determined effort waiting its moment to arise in the breasts of females seeking equality and unified activity in collective agreements.

Love will have its recognition through advancing further understandings of contained female energy. Womanhood will have its say, promoting true expression, through instigating female themes into the mainstays of communal affairs, which are embroidered skeins of wisdom and beauty with grace and style present in the woven tapestry.

We are involved in taking the reins of Divine Womanhood and delivering the female design of the Great Mother energy to those who are moved and ready to listen. We are not part of any movement such as ME TOO or any other feminine intimations or imitations of female energy. Please be cognisant when we say there is no other grouping of people with the understandings and information that we are programmed to take to the world, care of the Angel involvement working at the behest of the Great Mother.

Some are close to realizing an appreciation of cosmic Love energy, but fall down because they have not yet fully closed the gap on past happenings in this life and still rely on a variety of belief patterns that only give temporary support.

Are you Prepared?

A benefit of communal effort is to be instigated globally by the development of a new female leadership to rearrange old world flagging dispositions. We look forward to assisting that situational happening come into position shortly. We remind each of you who are listening that you have an interesting role to play. That role as you are quite aware has not yet been fully declared or clarified. So keep working on clearing waste residue from yourselves. Clean out dysfunctional areas of your ego system still carrying lingering pain from past practices.

How beautiful will the blossoms be that appear with the New Day when they first break into bloom. Understand that when the roses we speak come into bloom, those who are complacent with their planetary shortcomings are going to find themselves bereft of future benefit. This is not the time to rest on past laurels. This Divine Womanhood work has only just begun and soon it will be in earnest.

The Rainbow Trail

The Rainbow Trail signifies the return journey Home indemnifying human heritage.

To walk the Rainbow Trail offers an experiential and exponential journey of self-recovery and discovery cosmically designed to establish worth as a means of recovery in joining with the energy of ME, the Great Mother. It is of particular benefit for women seeking to locate certainty in their understanding of female status in a newly staged arena of Divine Womanhood development. Joy becomes available with the knowing of who you are and having a greater awareness of the life you are destined to realize.

The Rainbow Trail is a mystical story of human endeavour told in four parts. It begins with a separation of two selves and concludes with making a full connection with the unification of inner resources.

The getting of wisdom and recognition of internal beauty supplies fresh energy in mind to release inherent pain and fear, ego type apparel that is no longer necessary to wear. The breaking down of time-honoured myth-takes removes much of the interferences of accident and illness from within the human system.

Life and living free is truly attainable by first finding the means of letting go through an acceptance of willingness within each being.

Our next book 'The Star Within' features the theme from the Divine Womanhood Series, 'The Rainbow Trail'. Please indicate if you have an interest in building a new world of greater understanding in Love and Intelligence in community and we will be happy to relay further information.

Being-in-Love

Lucifer states clearly with each brother
'We have always been for you, Mother
Not even wisdom, nor beauty, nor joys
Can bring forth a bracelet of charms
These are toys, empty shells, merely ploys
If we have not entered within your arms
Death holds no purpose for souls sown wild
Who must we be when we cannot be your child

Where should we live if we do not dwell within thee
Where is our future if we do not combine with ME

This world doesn't carry a future above
It is a shroud holding people in thrall
People don't know yet of Beings-in-Love
And thus cannot commit to the All
We who these many lifetimes have strove
In showing worth must answer the call

www.ingramcontent.com/pod-product-compliance
Lightning Source LLC
Chambersburg PA
CBHW031415290426
44110CB00011B/387